WHEN CANCER COMES

by
CLARENCE McCONKEY

THE WESTMINSTER PRESS
PHILADELPHIA

PUBLISHED BY THE WESTMINSTER PRESS
®

PHILADELPHIA, PENNSYLVANIA

PRINTED IN THE UNITED STATES OF AMERICA

Library of Congress Cataloging in Publication Data

McConkey, Clarence.
    When cancer comes.

    Bibliography: p.
    1. Cancer. 2. Cancer patients. I. Title.
[DNLM: 1. Neoplasms—Popular works.
QZ201 M129w 1974]
RC263.M15   616.9′94   74–1330
ISBN 0–664–24987–6

WHEN
CANCER
COMES

To the Cancer Family:
Those who suffer, and their loved ones,
and
Those in the healing ministries

CONTENTS

INTRODUCTION

THIS IS A BOOK ABOUT CANCER. It is a book about the cancer patient, about the friends and family of the cancer patient, about research, diagnosis, and treatment of cancer, with some things about future projections. It contains some historical background about this disease, which is so prevalent everywhere. It speaks of the responses we make to cancer, of our individual uses of its note of adversity, and of some hope to which every person has a right. It is a book designed to be of help to, and to provide information for, the cancer sufferer today and to the literally millions of family members and friends who are touched by the lives and suffering of cancer patients everywhere.

This book is not in any sense a medical textbook. It is not intended to be a comprehensive treatment of the subject of cancer. It is written for the average person who understands very little about the complicated scientific language and procedures in the treatment of the disease but who I think is hungry for some sort of concise and easily understood information. The book is not written to provide easy answers to perplexing questions, to take lightly profound predicaments, nor to offer any false promise or cheap hope. It presents the possibility of hope, but that hope is carefully defined. Religion is an important ingredient in what I write, but this book is not founded on religious absolutes. Whether one is a Catholic, a Protestant, or a Jew, whether a skeptic or an atheist, is not an issue here. Cancer is not sectarian, and it does not pass over the believer.

It is my conviction that each person who reads this book will immediately understand that he is a member of what I choose to call the Cancer Family. Readers will know they belong to the body of human souls who make up this Family. This family relationship is established in one of three ways. First of all, many readers of this book will be bearers of cancer. They are thus patients and their membership in the Family is established by virtue of that fact. Wherever that cancer may be located in the body, whatever may be the present or future prognosis of the condition, however low the spirit or high the hope, this member of the Family is the one who has cancer and his membership in the Family is sustained in this way.

Secondly, the reader may be one of the members of the patient's family or he may be a close relative or a beloved friend. He sees the work of cancer in the patient dear to him. Free of the disease himself, he nevertheless enters into that bond of suffering established between persons when one of those persons suffers. That reader may be husband or father, mother or wife, child or parent. He may be brother or sister or pastor. Whatever the relationship within a human family or within the brotherhood of persons, there is suffering at work—that which comes when one member suffers for another. This is vicarious suffering and it is the suffering of the heart. Vicarious suffering has been written about and explained for centuries, but one must enter into the experience for himself to know how deep and traumatic the experience can be. In the Cancer Family we see again and again that suprahuman strain of love which would make one person quite willing to take upon himself the suffering of another if that were possible. Parents everywhere would suffer in place of their suffering child if some means were possible to transfer that suffering. Husbands and wives would gladly make that transfer. The fact that no such transfer of suffering can be made only highlights the intensity of the anguish that in fact does take place when one member of the Family suffers mentally because of the pain endured physically by another.

The third group of members of the Cancer Family are those persons in the healing professions: physicians, nurses, technicians, researchers, scientists, and clergymen. However unrelated these persons may be to the individual cancer patient, they are not in any way isolated from the Cancer Family. On their work, their concern, their skill and sympathy, hangs the thread of life and death for countless persons who are now suffering from cancer or who will suffer from cancer in the future. These persons take their calling seriously, and, while they enter into the Family in a somewhat oblique way, they are always included in Family gatherings. On one occasion I heard a noted surgeon say that the involvement of the physician in the collected sufferings of one day's experience in the hospital was more than enough to humanize him. The physician is a man who feels deeply the fact of suffering, and he in no wise wishes to abstain from active membership in the Family.

Well, what is the common bond that holds this Family together? The common bond is physical suffering. Much of that suffering lies within the body, the thought processes and emotions of the patient. We hurt in our bodies.

There is pain in the experience of cancer and that pain is felt deeply in bones, tissues, and organs. Yet not all the suffering within the membership of the Cancer Family is physical. There are undulations in the terrain of suffering. The cancer patient knows quite well the mental anguish that comes to family members, and he endures his share of that anguish. The patient suffers from loneliness and isolation. Chemotherapy can wash away diseased and dead cells, but it cannot wash away the pain of separation from loved ones which comes to settle in the distance between hospital and home. Physical pain is perhaps the most feared effect of cancer, but it is hardly the only effect.

The coming of cancer often brings about a new world for both patient and loved one. In that new world new perspectives are sometimes discovered. Time is suddenly found for things for which there was no time previously. Old things are often given up with little resistance. New things are taken on in stride. How easily we adjust to the necessities of the moment! Things that seemed eternal and indestructible are sometimes seen to be only transient. Things and relationships that formerly had only passing meaning for us suddenly become the object or relationship of supreme value. In this brotherhood there is uncertainty, but there is also new assurance of things of which the present only hints. How tremendous is the ability of men and women, young people and children, to see the importance of important things in this Family.

I share the intimacy of this Cancer Family with you. In that sense we are brothers across the time and distance that separates us. I share my concern for you and I suffer with you in your suffering. The disease which swept away that beautiful woman who was my wife, the disease of which I am now freed, makes us kin.

I am indebted to a number of persons in the writing of this book. Officials of the American Cancer Society were very kind in supplying me with information and materials. Two skilled staff members of Gorgas Hospital, Canal Zone, provided guidance in the writing of two of the sections. Dr. Henry Stockwell of the Department of Pediatrics made helpful suggestions and corrections in the section on cell structure. Dr. Harold Smith of the Department of Radiology read and made many important corrections in the section on radiotherapy. I appreciate their help immensely. I owe a special note of thanks to my secretary, Mrs. Ruth Auble, and to Mrs. Anne Marie Andersen for their typing skills. Joel must receive a word of appreciation for his help in proofreading. This book was at all times a joint effort of many persons, although I bear the responsibility for its lacks. Staff members in the medical library of Gorgas Hospital were helpful at all times and I owe them this word of appreciation and thanks.

Chapter 1

WHAT IS CANCER?

CANCER IS A DISEASE that is very likely as old as life itself. Signs of cancer have been found in the bones of animals that lived millions of years ago. It is found today in some form in every kind of living thing from plants and animals to man. It appears in many forms and under nearly every condition. It appears in many different ways under differing geographical, climatic, and environmental conditions. The ancient Egyptians knew about cancer and treated it with ointments, prayers, and spells. As remedies in the treatment of the disease, these were little improved on until the nineteenth century. Because the ancient Greeks, another people knowledgeable about medical and scientific phenomena, thought that spreading cancerous growths resembled the claws of a crab, they called it the crablike disease, *karkinos*.[1] The Latin translation of the word was *cancer*, and that is the name we commonly use for this disease. Anyone who has ever seen a color plate of an advanced malignant tumor will notice the resemblance between the spreading tentacles of the tumor and the figure of the crab. An octupus also comes to mind when we see the long arms of such a tumor.

There is in existence today an ancient document

called the Ebers papyrus, written approximately 1550
B.C. This document is a compilation of traditional Egyp-
tian medical knowledge and treatment, a kind of medical textbook, so to speak. In this papyrus there is a
description of a type of cancer known to medical science
today, with comments, incantations, and prayers to be
said when preparing or using certain medicines prescribed for that cancer. This document is one of many
that provide knowledge about ancient responses to, and
inquiry into, the disease of cancer. Man has been actively
fighting cancer since it was identified medically in the
time of the great Greek physician Hippocrates, the
father of modern medicine, about 400 B.C. Forms and
methods used in that fight have sometimes been strange
and varied, but they are to be appreciated nevertheless
for the light they shed on the disease through the ages.

Types of cancer that afflict human beings are classified today by medical science in several different ways.
Some workers in the field of cancer research and treatment list four basic types of cancer. There are others who
identify the disease according to three basic types. If one
uses the lowest common denominator in classifying cancer, it is possible to classify it according to two categories determined by the tissues of the body in which
they arise.

The medical term for the first of these is carcinoma.
Carcinomas are cancers originating in epithelial tissue,
such as the skin or lining of the colon, lung, womb,
breast, prostate, etc. In this sense carcinomas are cancers
found in the organs of the body. The second basic type of
cancer is sarcoma. Sarcomas are cancers arising from or
originating in connective or supportive tissues such as
bone, cartilage, or muscle. These are cancers arising in
nonepithelial tissue. If we add a third type of cancer

here, it would be that of the family of leukemia-lymphoma cancers. These are cancers arising in bone marrow and lymph nodes. Generically it is possible to include these latter cancers among the sarcomas, but the leukemia-lymphoma cancers are such distinctive cancers —or neoplasms, as cancers are referred to medically— that it is sometimes helpful to see them separately. New forms of cancer are identified periodically, but they continue to be classified according to present typings.

Perhaps the greatest enigma of the whole field of cancer research, detection, and treatment is the question concerning the origins and causes of cancer. What is it exactly that brings on this destructive malady? What is its cause or beginning? How do we account for it? Those are questions which have a variety of answers, some of them specific ones, some of them only general ones. It is not really possible to say that cancer is caused by a certain thing or even by a certain combination of things in most cases. We will see in a moment that it is possible to pinpoint the moment when cancer begins in the human body even though we never know when that moment actually occurs. At the same time it is just as difficult to deny that cancer is caused by a thing or things that are rather clearly identified presently. We know quite a lot about many aspects of cancer-causing agents—or carcinogens, as they are called—and the relationship between those agents and the presence of cancer seems pretty clear in many cases. Perhaps the most notable example of this is the relationship between lung cancer and cigarette smoking. It is of course entirely possible to claim that lung cancer is caused by factors *other* than cigarette smoking or by factors *in addition* to cigarette smoking. But there is such a weight of evidence pointing in the direction of a direct lung cancer–cigarette smoking relationship that one is hard pressed to deny the conclusions drawn by the medical scientist. In January, 1964, the Surgeon General of the United States said:

> Cigarette smoking is causally related to lung cancer in men; the magnitude of the effect . . . far outweighs all other factors. The data for women, though less extensive, point in the same direction. The risk of developing lung cancer increases with duration of smoking and the number of cigarettes smoked per day, and is diminished by discontinuing.[2]

This report was based on the findings of doctors and scientists engaged in long-range research. A body of responsible evidence that has been accumulated since the report was published has served to substantiate the original conclusion. For this reason it is possible for the medical scientist to say that cigarette smoking causes lung cancer. This is not to say that *all* lung cancer is caused by cigarette smoking or that cigarette smoking *always* results in lung cancer. However, the death rate from lung cancer in cigarette smokers is about ten times that of nonsmokers. It is estimated that 75 percent of lung cancer is caused by smoking. At the present time most cases of lung cancer are incurable. The life expectancy of a two-pack-a-day smoker at age twenty-five is 8.3 years less than that of a nonsmoker. A heavy cigarette smoker's chances of dying during his prime are almost twice as great as a nonsmoker's.[3] In 1972, 72,000 persons died of lung cancer in the United States, and current projections show an increase in this figure for 1974.

There are other cancers that also have generally well defined single causes. Overexposure to the sun is a well-known cause of many forms of skin cancer. Sun-induced carcinomas nearly always remain malignancy-free when the sun factor is reduced or removed. A high-density exposure to radiation is known to be a prime agent in the development of leukemia in many persons whose leukemia can be traced to overexposure to radiation.

Beyond these rather well defined cancer-causing relationships we are not at the present time able to establish with certainty the causes of cancer. It remains to be determined just what agent or combination of agents or conditions in the body and in the environment produce the cell structure changes that give rise to the cancerous condition. Suspected causes are well known. Certain factors in heredity seem to play a part in the conditions of the body that favor the growth of cancer. Medical science holds that certain genetically inherited traits or weaknesses may cause certain forms of cancer to follow familiar patterns. Breast cancer is one example of this. By this I mean that there are certain correlations between mothers and daughters who have breast cancer that seem to suggest a genetically related factor. The aging process, such as that affecting the onset of prostatic cancer in men, is another example of something that is tied into the genetic makeup of the human being. Chronic irritation of a section of skin or tissue has been found to be a factor in the presence of cancer in that tissue. Viruses are known to be directly associated with the development of certain cancers, and viruses are a major focal point of research today. Pollutants in the atmosphere, such as toxic fumes from industrial wastes and automobile exhaust fumes, as well as occupational pollutants such as asbestos dust, coal dust, and cement residues, are additional agents known to have an influence on the development of some cancers. Some dietary factors, such as the absence of certain nutrients or an oversupply of those nutrients, also come into focus in our study of cancer-producing agents. Injuries to bones or tissues, and the whole field of personality or character traits, are other factors in the repertoire of cancer-causing or cancer-influencing agents. To what extent any of these factors or agents is the direct cause of cancer in any particular person is nearly impossible to determine at the present time because of our lack of knowledge about so many aspects of cancer. We do know that certain relationships do exist between them and cancer, and those relationships are currently under intensive study.

Chapter 2

WHO GETS CANCER?

THE QUESTION as to *who* gets cancer is also an imperfectly answered question. Is there a cancer-susceptible person, one who might well represent the general *profile* of a cancer-prone person in general? To a certain extent the answer to this is, Yes! While cancer cuts across all known lines of age, condition, and circumstances, we do know some things about the general profile of the disease and the patient who gets the disease. It is possible in this way to achieve some general idea of who *might* get cancer, or who might have a better chance of *not* getting cancer than others. By a study of family background, of occupation, dietary habits, the smoking record and other factors in the life of any person, the medical scientist can draw some conclusions about the cancer-prone profile of an individual. This requires an extensive amount of information and analysis of that information, but it is entirely possible that the time will come when any adult will be able to have a "cancer diagnostic check" to determine his likelihood of having a particular form of cancer. In the meantime we can only see what the picture of cancer is like by viewing the statistics.

It is estimated that 53,000,000 Americans now living, or one in four, will eventually have cancer in some form and to some degree.[4] This will be true unless there is some dramatic and immediate breakthrough in cancer-prevention knowledge. Barring that possibility, we know that cancer will strike over the years in approximately two of every three American families. In the decade of the 1970's there will be an estimated 3,500,000 cancer deaths, 6,500,000 new cancer cases, and more than 10,000,000 cancer patients under medical care in the United States. Cancer strikes all ages and nationalities. Infants are sometimes born badly afflicted with cancer. It affects children as well as adults, but it strikes with increasing frequency with advancing age. Approximately 1,000,000 persons will be treated for cancer in the United States in 1974. Approximately 655,000 new cancer cases will be diagnosed. In 1973 an estimated 349,000 Americans died of cancer. In 1974 about 355,000 persons will die of cancer in the United States. That is the equivalent of about 975 persons a day, or one every one and one half minutes. Of every six deaths from all causes in this country, one is from cancer.

Cancer is the leading cause of death among women, ages thirty to fifty-four. More than half of all cancer deaths are among persons over sixty-five years of age. In recent years more men than women have died of cancer. It is anticipated that the ratio in 1974 will be about 54 to 46. In 1974 cancer will take the lives of approximately 3,500 children under the age of fifteen. Almost half of those children will die of acute leukemia, a cancer of the blood-forming tissues. More school children die of cancer than from any other disease. Today there are over 300,000 American children under eighteen who have lost their fathers to cancer. Over 250,000 have lost their mothers. Multiply these figures the world over and the number becomes so enormous it staggers the imagination.

In 1974 approximately 32,500 women will die of breast cancer in the United States. Surprisingly, 250 men will die of breast cancer. About 1,800 persons will die of cancer of the tongue. An estimated 19,400 persons will die of pancreatic cancer, a form of cancer that is spiraling upward statistically each year for reasons not yet known. In 1974 approximately 19,000 men and 22,800 women will die of cancer of the genital organs. Approximately 15,300 persons will die of leukemia.

One of the most perplexing factors in cancer research and treatment is that related to certain geographical differences in the incidence of cancer and the rate of deaths from cancer. Some of these differences may be seen in death rate statistics for the United States. We know that Alaska, for example, has the lowest death rate for cancer among the fifty states. We do not really know why. The current (1974) projected cancer death rate in that northernmost state is 62 deaths per 100,000 population. Maine currently has the highest projected cancer death rate in the nation, 212 per 100,000 population, followed by Rhode Island (204), West Virginia (201), New York (200), and the District of Columbia (199). State by state the 1974 estimated number of deaths and the death rate per 100,000 population is as shown in the table on page 24.[5]

As startling as these statistics from the United States may be, they are hardly more so than those gathered from around the world. In a fairly recent statistical comparison of 40 countries,[6] Scotland ranked number one in cancer deaths from all causes for males, with 201.4 deaths per 100,000 population. Czechoslovakia was

State	Number of Deaths	Death Rate per 100,000 Population
Alabama	5,400	155
Alaska	200	62
Arizona	2,600	134
Arkansas	3,500	175
California	33,200	153
Colorado	2,900	122
Connecticut	5,400	167
Delaware	900	152
District of Columbia	1,600	199
Florida	14,600	197
Georgia	6,300	130
Hawaii	900	110
Idaho	1,100	150
Illinois	19,900	172
Indiana	8,600	158
Iowa	5,200	182
Kansas	4,000	175
Kentucky	5,400	165
Louisiana	5,900	156
Maine	2,200	212
Maryland	6,400	150
Massachusetts	11,200	189
Michigan	14,500	155
Minnesota	6,500	163
Mississippi	3,600	162
Missouri	8,900	184
Montana	1,300	185
Nebraska	2,800	185
Nevada	750	133
New Hampshire	1,500	189
New Jersey	14,000	184
New Mexico	1,200	115
New York	37,700	200
North Carolina	6,900	132
North Dakota	1,100	181
Ohio	19,000	172

State	Number of Deaths	Death Rate per 100,000 Population
Oklahoma	4,500	170
Oregon	3,700	166
Pennsylvania	23,500	197
Rhode Island	2,000	204
South Carolina	3,500	132
South Dakota	1,200	182
Tennessee	6,300	155
Texas	17,100	144
Utah	1,100	97
Vermont	850	182
Virginia	6,800	139
Washington	5,600	154
West Virginia	3,400	201
Wisconsin	7,800	169
Wyoming	500	149

second highest at 195.7, followed by Austria at 192.2. Nicaragua had the lowest death rate for males at 22.0, followed by Thailand at 22.2. Scotland has the highest death rate for cancer of the colon and rectum in males. In lung cancer Scotland ranked number one for males and number two for females. Nicaragua had the lowest death rates, for both males and females for oral cancer (cancer of the mouth and surrounding tissues), cancer of the colon and rectum, and lung cancer. El Salvador, Nicaragua's next-door neighbor, ranked 38th for males, and 37th for females in deaths from cancer in all sites; 39th for both males and females in deaths from lung cancer. Thailand had the lowest death rate for cancer of the skin in females, cancer of the prostate in males, and leukemia in both men and women. It ranked 39th for cancer of the colon and rectum in females, breast and uterus cancer, skin cancer in males, and stomach cancer in both male and females. Why Thailand had such an overall low death rate is something the scientist is asking and pondering.

Chile and Denmark shared the grim distinction of having the highest death rate for cancer in women of all the countries surveyed, both reporting a death rate of 138.8 per 100,000 population. Austria ranked third highest for cancer deaths of women, with 130. The lowest rates were reported by Nicaragua, which ranked 39th with a rate of 37.3, and Thailand, which ranked 40th with only 14.6 deaths per 100,000.

In all these geographical areas there are factors at work such as climate, diet, ecology, environment, and personal hygiene. Much research must be done before we are able to draw binding conclusions about the meaning of the data. Time will tell what it all means. In the meanwhile we must live with the certain knowledge that cancer is a product of man's environment, of his genetic makeup, and of other factors not yet understood or even known. Only as we approach these factors with complete scientific analysis will cancer be more fully understood and eliminated from the experience of man.

Chapter 3

HOW CANCER BEGINS

THE HUMAN BODY, the focal point of all our discussion about cancer, is a mighty wondrous piece of creation. It has been described, analyzed, poeticized, sculptured, painted, extolled, and profaned. The body is at once pampered and abused. It is the source of our bodily pleasures and all our pain. It is the place of our greatest virtues and our grossest iniquities. It provides us enormous joy and indescribable sadness. The body is filled with love's capacities and hate's possibilities. It is the place of the spirit, the home of the soul, the seat of the mind. It has room for exquisite tenderness and for unlimited bitterness. The body is light as well as darkness. It knows the first cry of life and the last whisper of death. It is the area of all wisdom and the "habitation of dragons." It is the home of all that makes us the human beings we are—emotions, motivations, sensations, and thoughts. The body is our earthly home and it is a many-mansioned edifice. It is the source of ceaseless wonder and unutterable mystery.

It is a complicated mechanism, this body of ours, a colossal system of things. About seven tenths of the adult human body is water. Since all life originated in or near the sea, it may be that this water content reflects something of our primordial ancestry. The body functions according to the working of its seven internal systems, digestive, urinary, respiratory, skeletal-muscular, circulatory, reproductive, and nervous. It has two glandular systems, exocrine and endocrine. The exocrine glands secrete fluids such as saliva, tears, sweat, bile, and mucus. The endocrine glands, for example, the pituitary, thyroid, and adrenal, secrete hormones. The human body contains twenty-five feet of intestine. It contains from ten to fourteen pints of blood, and the human heart beats about seventy-two times per minute in order to pump that blood through the labyrinth of arteries, vessels, and capillaries that fill the body. It has a blood vessel system so long that if all the vessels were laid end to end, it would make a line stretching 100,000 miles, or four times around the earth. The body is a wonderfully timed mechanism, providing the means by which systems and processes begin, function, and end at the proper moments day after day for efficient operation. The body is directed by an intricate and not fully understood brain mechanism. No two human bodies are alike, all of them having different characteristics of appearance, size, and emotional makeup, to say nothing of differences of hand and foot prints. The body works like a machine in many important ways, but it is vastly more complicated and intricate than a machine. It stands perhaps as the epitome of what the theologian wishes to call the "acts of creation."

The key to the creation and sustaining of all life is the reproductive system. Reproduction takes place, in one sense, when the male sperm and female egg are united in the female of higher forms of life. When sperm and egg unite, a new organism is created. This is reproduction of the species. All normally developed human bodies have reproductive organs. We are reproducing creatures. Once sperm and egg have united in the womb of the female, there begins another kind of reproduction. The newly created organism, initially a one-celled being, begins to divide, or to reproduce itself. It breaks apart so to speak, becomes two cells, and we then have the beginning of the process of mitosis. Without hesitation these cells divide and become four cells, and soon these four become eight as mitosis continues. This process of cell division is the key to growth, and it continues throughout the life-span of every living creature. That process ceases only when the body dies. The initial division of the cell created by union of sperm and egg is but the beginning of the creation of an astronomical number of cells in the lifetime of the organism.

The body of a mature man has more than a trillion (1,000,000,000,000) cells. Every minute about three billion cells in our bodies die, and in that same time about three billion new cells are born. Cells in different parts of the body live for varying lengths of time, however. A white blood cell lives for about thirteen days and a liver cell about eighteen months. A nerve cell can live for a hundred years. Red blood cells, on the other hand, may die at the rate of two million per second. All the potential of a human body, its sex, shape, color, size, and functioning, is determined by the cell structure system contained in the single cell created by union of sperm and egg. Within each cell there is a complex chemical substance called DNA (deoxyribonucleic acid), the wondrous structure of which has only recently been discovered. The way in which DNA is responsible for the process of cell division and how it guides that process is a very intricate and complicated subject. We understand that DNA is present in the chromosomes, those microscopic, spindle-like particles which are the genetic materials that carry all the instructions and directions for the development of the new living organism. DNA is the brain system through which the chromosomes form the shape of the new living entity. It tells the cells being produced which of them will be bone cells and which blood cells, muscle cells, or internal organ cells. DNA is called "the master plan of life." There are other factors and processes that guide the development of the new living creature, but DNA is the key to it all. DNA is present in the genetic structure of the cell at the moment of conception, provided by parent cells in sperm and egg, and it guides the development of the fetus and the growth of the resultant body throughout the lifetime of that body. It continues to function until death overtakes that body and all bodily processes cease. Then, and only then, does DNA cease to function.

Just as there would be no continuation of the species if male and female could not unite to form a new living creature, or if the one-celled creature produced by the union of sperm and egg did not divide to make two cells, so would there be no continuation of life if that cell division, or mitosis, did not continue throughout the life-span of the human being created. That process of cell division is the key to the continuation of every species. Our understanding of that process is also the key to our understanding of cancer.

The rate of cell division within the human body is set within the first moments of life following conception. That rate is rapid in the first years of life, and of necessity during this time more cells are born than die. This is why the body grows. Body growth is simply the addition of cells to the structure of the body. In infancy more cells are born than die. As we move toward physical maturity the DNA factor in us provides for about the same number of cells to die as are born. In other words, the rate of cell division slows down or evens out. This is the way in which mature physical size is maintained. In later life more cells die than are born. This is one cause of body decline in aging. Each organ, each tissue, each system has its own cell division timing mechanism. If the rate of cell division were not carefully timed, an eight-month-old infant would weigh as much as the earth. This is prevented by the enormous death rate of cells. DNA sets the timing for cell birth and for cell death in every single cell of the body. This check-and-balance system in cell division is the key to normal development in the human body. Cells divide at the right time, in the right way, and in the right number, according to inherited genetic guidelines determined by DNA. In the great majority of cases this cell division takes place on time and in the manner prescribed by DNA, and the process goes on throughout life.

Sometimes, however, this check-and-balance system fails. Just as we do not yet fully understand the working of DNA, nor the larger cell division and "code of life" process, so do we not yet fully understand the reasons behind the failure of the cell division process to proceed on schedule, the reasons why it does something different. When the cell division process does not act in the prescribed way we know that somewhere, in some way, the genetic controls have been thrown off. In that process one cell may become three or four instead of two. The multiplication rate may be speeded up. What we see then is the creation of too many cells for the particular bone or organ. We have runaway cells—mavericks, you might say—which do not act in the ways prescribed for the cells of that bone or organ. They do not respond to the check-and-balance system. These wild cells may lose their customary shapes and forms and take on irregular shapes different from those of the parent or surrounding cells.

These aberrant cells do not function as the surrounding cells function. Actually they are functionless, cells without purpose, although they are active cells. Their activity is the problem. These cells multiply and begin to interfere with the normal cells, crowding in, around, and through the cell structure of the organ or bone until something is smothered, overpowered, and wounded. Then the bodily processes begin to break down.

The question is, What causes this wild growth of cells? That question, together with its answer, is the key to our whole understanding of cancer. Once we know the answer to that question, or at least understand the question in a better way, we will probably know how to prevent cancer and how to treat it effectively if it begins. Our present knowledge leading to an answer is very limited and incomplete. However, we do know some things about the causes of this wild growth. Present in the cell structure of the human body is another chemical factor called RNA (ribonucleic acid). RNA is like a messenger that carries out the orders of DNA. DNA says that this cell will be a red-hair-producing cell and RNA rushes out to make sure that the cell produces a red hair. But sometimes an outside force exerts pressure on RNA to become insubordinate, to give orders rather than to take orders. When that happens, at that precise moment the conditions are created for an abnormal cell activity to start that may result in cancer. What pressure causes RNA to thwart the good intentions of DNA? Somehow the influences we have already mentioned—heredity, diet, irritation of a tissue, a virus, etc.—seem to provide the clue to this thwarting of the beneficial work of DNA. These influences, one or more of them, produce some kind of conflict between DNA and RNA, and when this happens RNA may simply override the orders of DNA, telling the cells in effect to multiply as rapidly as they wish, anytime they wish, in any way they wish. Much of the research in the field of cancer today is being done in the area of viruses in an attempt to understand more fully the makeup and workings of viral and other possible cancer-causing influences upon the cell structure. Certainly we are safe in saying that cancer begins in the human body at that precise moment when the DNA-ordered and controlled process of cell division, or mitosis, is somehow interfered with and orders are received from some other source by the cells, telling them to divide as they wish without controls. When that moment occurs, a human body may become cancerous.

Chapter 4

PREVENTION
AND TREATMENT

IT IS NOT POSSIBLE at the present time to detect the precise moment when, through some disturbance of the controlled process of mitosis, cancer begins somewhere in the body of a person. Therefore we must depend on our knowledge of detection, prevention, and treatment to control that newly arisen cancer. When the diagnosis is finally made that cancer is indeed present, the physician begins to decide what response he will make in his effort to fight the malignancy. He will not offer any unproven promises of cancer cure. However, from the outset of this discussion we will want to remember that persons are cured of cancer every day in treatment centers around the world. The term "cured" has special meaning for us here. In general, with reference to cancer, medical science defines "cured" as the condition of being free of any active form of cancer for a period of five years after the conclusion of the treatment process. In the United States approximately 218,000 persons will be saved from cancer in 1974. At the present time a total of 1,500,000 Americans are classified as being cured of cancer. It almost always comes as a surprise when people learn that cancer is one of the most curable of our major diseases. There is every reason to believe that the rate of cancer cure will continue to rise through the development of more sophisticated methods of treatment and additional discoveries about its nature and its causes. We are not being naïve at all when we say that, in the midst of the mortality statistics regarding cancer, there is an abundance of statistical evidence to show the life-supporting nature of cancer treatment. In my experiences with cancer over the years I am more and more impressed, not with the number of persons who die from cancer, but with the number of persons who continue to live after having had cancer.

The most fundamental approach to the treatment of cancer is the prevention of cancer, and it is at this point we begin our discussion. We begin with the basic fact that one has no need to be treated for what he does not have. For this reason there is literally no way to over-emphasize the importance of prevention knowledge and method. It is now estimated by the American Cancer Society that as many as 100,000 persons who will eventually die of cancer could have avoided cancer altogether, or been saved from cancer, if detection had taken place earlier. Detection of cancer in its early stages is a form of preventive medicine. This prevention through detection is possible not only through various examination techniques that the physician may use in making regular and special physical checkups but also through the knowledge of cancer's warning signs on the part of each individual. In addition, many persons who have developed cancer and eventually died of cancer could have been kept free of cancer in the beginning if certain preventive measures had been followed. We have already touched on the causal relationship between cancer of the lung and cigarette smoking. There seems little reason to doubt the word of medical science that great numbers of persons who die of lung cancer would never have had lung cancer if they had not smoked cigarettes or if they had stopped smoking before the onset of cancer. Many persons who suffer from cancer of the skin might very well have escaped that sometimes dangerous form of cancer entirely had they not absorbed excessive amounts of sunlight. A sore that does not heal, a bruise that is periodically reinjured but not attended to, untreated hemorrhoids—these are situations in the human body that may turn cancerous through neglect. Treated, these conditions are normally noncancerous for long periods of time, and may be completely eliminated as a source of future trouble. Untreated, they may very well, and often do, develop into cancerous tissue. Prevention in so many cases may mean the difference between cancer and no cancer, between a benign tumor being eliminated or its finally turning malignant, between being cancerous and of being cancer-free. In a word, prevention may well mean the difference between life and death.

It would be impossible here to describe in any detail the many preventive techniques and procedures available to us today. They range all the way from simple observation of a sore or lump to the medical use of complicated machinery. In their most basic form, prevention methods are those put into use by individuals in the privacy of their own homes. I will suggest to you those simple but crucial signs so familiar to us all—cancer's seven warning signals:

1. Change in bowel or bladder habits
2. A sore that does not heal
3. Unusual bleeding or discharge
4. Thickening or lump in breast or elsewhere

  5. Indigestion or difficulty in swallowing
  6. Obvious change in wart or mole
  7. Nagging cough or hoarseness

The discovery of any one of these conditions in our bodies followed by an appointment with a physician is the primary method of prevention.

Women have available to them two important techniques of cancer prevention. These two techniques involve the detection of cancer in the two most vulnerable areas of the woman's body, the breasts and the uterus. Detection of either cancer or a precancerous condition in the breasts often takes place at the point of a woman's examination of her own breasts. In spite of the fact that any woman can give herself frequent breast self-examinations, and that a physician can do this in a matter of minutes, there are great numbers of women who are not familiar with the procedures of such self-examination. We cannot forget that 90,000 new cases of breast cancer and 33,000 deaths from breast cancer are anticipated in 1974. At present rates, one of every 15 American women will some day develop breast cancer. Many women now doomed could be kept cancer-free if they would be more knowledgeable of, and careful about, cancer's warnings. There is little question among medical scientists that the death rate for breast cancer in women could be significantly reduced if more women practiced self-examination of the breasts regularly, and if they submitted to an examination by a physician more frequently. The earlier the detection of breast cancer, the greater the chances that it can be treated successfully. There is an 85 percent chance of survival for five years or longer when breast cancer is treated before it spreads to other organs or tissues through the process of metastasis. This is possible with early detection. Between 65 and 80 percent of biopsies of lumps in the breast are found to be benign. To find tumors in this state and to have them treated or removed permits the expectation that continued long life will follow. To wait until the benign tumor has become malignant is to invite prolonged suffering and possible death.

A second basic tool available to women for preventive purposes is the Pap test. This test is standard procedure for nearly all physicians today. Through this test a cancerous or precancerous condition of the uterine area can be detected and treated before there is an enlargement or spreading of the condition. The Pap test is a process of scraping the uterine area and analyzing the "smear," or gathered scrapings, in the laboratory. As simple and routine as this procedure is, there is still widespread neglect of the test by great numbers of women. It is certain that if more women would have more frequent Pap smears as a part of their normal physical care, the rate of uterine cancer could be dramatically reduced. There is now the possibility that sometime soon a do-it-yourself Pap smear kit will be available for home use by women.

Use of the proctoscope is another preventive technique now employed by many physicians. The proctoscope, or procto, as it is commonly called, is a lighted tube inserted by the physician through the rectal opening into the lower part of the colon. With light flooding the colon the physician can detect any growths or abnormalities in this cancer-prone section of the body. While this technique is perhaps a bit untidy or an embarrassment to some persons, the proctoscope is a marvelous instrument and contributes greatly to early detection of

rectal cancer. Any person can ask for the procto examination if it is not offered voluntarily by the physician.

Just now coming into use is a procedure known as
liquid crystal (L.C.) thermography. This is a procedure
by which the trained physician or technician can measure
the temperature of a tissue or gland as a clue to the
presence of cancer. At the present time this method is not
100 percent foolproof, but it gives promise of greater
future success, especially in the detection of cancer of the
breast. The time may very well come when liquid crystal
thermography can be given to females with as much ease
as the Pap test. If this proves to be true, detection of
cancer of the breast will receive an enormous boon.

Another method of cancer prevention through detection is that of examination of the female cervix by means
of an instrument called the cytoanalyzer. This instrument
makes it possible to scan electronically screening smears
of the cervix. It goes beyond the capacities of the Pap
test although it complements that basic procedure in
detection of cancerous cells in the uterus.

The xeroradiograph is one of many machines or instruments now being used in the general field of mammography. Several techniques exist by which the trained
physician or technician can electronically scan or view
the tissues of the human body, especially the female
breast. This is generally what mammography is about.
There are other prevention-through-detection techniques
in use at present. For example, it was found in a survey
of 4,800 women between the ages of thirty-five and
fifty-five that women with early carcinomas of the breast
excrete subnormal amounts of urinary metabolites of
androgen and cortisol. Through the examination of urine
specimens it might very well be possible to detect the
presence of breast carcinoma long before it can be seen

visually or felt by either the person or a physician.[7] The number of women involved in the survey described would seem to justify the conclusion of the authors that this technique of urinary analysis gives great promise for the future detection of breast cancer.

These tests, instruments, and examination techniques are but a few of the growing number of procedures available to the physician in cancer detection and prevention. The list continues to grow, and more and more we come under the influence of the results of research of past years in all these areas. Rather swiftly, I suspect, we will see significant new advances in detection and prevention procedures, and as this happens we will see a steady decline in the rate of new cancer growth and in the rate of cancer death. This is a prospect to be warmly welcomed, and when it comes about we will need to reward those scientists, physicians, technicians, and workers in the fields of cancer research and treatment who have made that achievement possible. The roll call will be long indeed.

For 655,000 persons living in the United States this prospect will not be enough. That is the number of new cancer cases that are anticipated in 1974. In those cases, and in other cases throughout the world in which cancer is diagnosed, there will need to be something more. That something more, of course, will be some form of treatment. To the scientific treatment of cancer we now move in this discussion.

The medical treatment of cancer today is fundamentally a science operating under a three-pronged approach. Once cancer is detected in the body all the resources available to medical science are made available to the patient. This ministry of medicine is not only available within a local hospital complex. It operates throughout an entire city hospital system as hospitals, laboratories, and universities share information, exchange opinions, and collaborate on diagnosis and treatment. In this exchange physicians are available to one another for consultation and advice. There is an even larger dimension to treatment than this. The cancer patient has available to him today the resources of hospitals, laboratories, research foundations, and medical personnel far from where he might live at any given time. A patient can be flown, for example, anywhere in the world to treatment facilities. How well I remember the boy in San José, Costa Rica, with a diagnosis of leukemia. The child was hospitalized in that Central American city for examination and treatment. Tests of bone marrow taken from the boy were flown to Houston, Texas, for examination. On the basis of the diagnosis, specialists in Houston recommended a treatment drug that was available at the Johns Hopkins University School of Medicine in Baltimore. A specialist in the field of leukemia from The New York Hospital flew to Baltimore to get the serum, went on to Houston to consult with laboratory and medical personnel involved in the testing, and with this information flew to Costa Rica as a consulting physician in the treatment of the boy. Such is the nature of a worldwide ministry of medical service available to the cancer patient today. This ministry now makes it possible for any physician in the world to have the certainty that he is a part of a program of healing with universal scope. He need no longer feel that he is isolated from the sources of specialized help and information.

Since cancer is not one but many diseases, it follows that treatment consists not of one method or approach but of many approaches. The treatment brought to bear upon any one patient is determined by that patient's need and condition. Depending on the site of the cancer, on its form and stage of advancement, the physician will respond to it with the methods that are appropriate and possible. We know there are over three hundred kinds of cancer. Some of these grow very rapidly, while others grow very slowly. Some types of cancer are always fatal at the present time, others are seldom fatal. Some respond to many kinds of treatment. Some respond to only one or two kinds. Some respond to none. Cancer affects persons differently in different parts of the world, as we have already seen. It affects persons under differing conditions. It is a deceitful enemy and our response to it must be as severe and aggressive as possible. In every way we must learn to outwit the enemy.

Medical science is doing a fair job of just that. In this section we will discover some facts about the three basic approaches to treatment of cancer, some of the newer forms just now coming into use, and what some of these forms mean to us today. These three basic forms are surgery, radiation, and chemotherapy.

The oldest and most frequently used method of cancer treatment is surgery. The science of surgery and the skill of the surgeon has been written about and described extensively in the literature of the world. Mostly this has been to the advantage of both medical science and the patient because some of the surgical techniques used by the physician became familiar to future patients. Surgery is performed today on nearly every section of the human body. While this does not mean that surgery necessarily can bring about change for the better in every part of the body, at least every section of the body can be exposed for study and examination. This often involves very localized kinds of cutting. Removal of a mole, opening of a surface lesion, cutting back a benign growth, can often take place in a doctor's office under very little anesthesia. Once this is done, the patient may go home and forget about the cutting.

Other surgery is more extensive. In that case it may involve removal of a mass in some part of the body, loss of an arm or foot, deep incisions in a muscle or organ. In such cases surgery is carried out by a surgical team working in a hospital operating room, and deep anesthesia is required. Recovery in such cases may require days or weeks, even months.

Surgery may involve radical cutting of the human body at one or many points. The names of the surgical techniques read like something from e. e. cummings or Ogden Nash. A mastectomy involves the removal of a breast. We normally associate this with the removal of the female breast, but mastectomy is also the surgical name for removal of the male breast in cases of cancer of the male breast gland. A laryngectomy is surgical removal of the entire larynx or voice box, as a result of which one loses his voice. Mechanical devices are now used that permit the patient to resume the practice of speaking again after speech rehabilitation. A lobectomy involves the removal of a lobe, e.g., of a lung, liver, or thyroid. A colostomy is the removal of a cancerous section of the large intestine and the rerouting of the elimination duct to a tube that extends out through the abdominal wall. Persons who have had a colostomy normally perform their elimination chores by the use of a bag that is worn strapped to the leg. As disagreeable as this procedure may seem at first glance, it is a lifesaver to thousands of persons who gladly put up with a minor inconvenience in exchange for life itself. A tracheostomy is the opening of the throat to the windpipe and the placement of a tube into the windpipe for either temporary or permanent breathing. A gastrostomy is the surgical placement of a tube into the stomach from outside the body in order to introduce food directly into the stomach, bypassing the normal route in the process of eating. An urethrostomy is the artificial tubal draining of the bladder. A thyroidectomy is the removal of the thyroid. Neck dissection is the removal of the lymph nodes on one or both sides of the neck, usually involving rather radical cutting. Prostatectomy is the surgical removal of the prostate in males. For a real example of the highly sophisticated terminology used by medical science today in surgery we will remember that a "hysterectomy with bilateral salpingo-oophorectomy" is the designation the physician uses for the removal of the female organs in the pelvic area. These are but a few of the terms used in the science of surgery and they are all part of our approach to cancer treatment.

We know, of course, that procedures and methods of surgery continue to be improved constantly. This increased proficiency in surgical techniques has come about simply because we learn more and more about the human body and how to treat it, more and more about cancer itself, and more about how to use surgical techniques in the fight against cancer. Improved means of controlling infections, more effective anesthetics, and wider use of blood substitutes are among the advancements related to surgery. We live in a time in which the skill of the surgeon plays an increasing part in the prolongation of human life, and it is the general conviction of all medical workers that we stand on the threshold of continued breathless breakthroughs in the science of surgery. Areas of the human body that have not been previously accessible to surgical techniques will become available in the future. Organs of the body that have not been receptive to surgical techniques (such as the pancreas) and organs that have not been transplantable in the past (such as the brain or the genitals) may very well become available to the surgeon for successful surgery as a result of more effective use of antibiotics, transplant antirejection drugs, and increased artificial regulation of the bodily processes. Much remains to be discovered in the field of surgery. But much that we have mentioned is available now to the cancer patient when he comes to his physician with cancer anywhere in the body. Surgical procedures are not the complete answer in any way, but they constitute a basic and vital approach.

The second major category of cancer treatment is irradiation. This is a general term used for a wide variety of methods that bring to bear on cancerous tissues the burning and killing rays of radiation. In its simplest form irradiation has as its function the burning up, shriveling, and eventual killing of cancer cells. The history of radiotherapy technique in the treatment of cancer is a rather brief one insofar as the history of medical science itself is concerned. The oldest of these techniques involved the use of radium. Treatment by radium was the first effective and consistently useful tool in the field of radiation treatment of cancer. Early use of this powerful element, an element derived from pitchblende ore, was sometimes as deadly to the patient as to the cancer, but more sophisticated management of its use led to significant results in later years. Radium is still an important factor in the field of radiotherapy but its use is more specialized and restricted than before. Radium continues to be used both in terms of direct exposure to cancerous tissues in the body and in implanted objects such as radium-charged needles and "bullets" buried deep in tissue or bone.

In the last ten years or so new forms of irradiation have been developed and put into general use that exceed the effectiveness of most radium treatments. Perhaps the most common term today among laymen in cancer treatment is "cobalt." This is not surprising, since cobalt therapy remains the basic means of treatment by radioactive elements. Cobalt is an element found in natural ores that bear nickel, iron, lead, copper, and zinc. It is a tough, silver-white metallic element in its natural state. As such it is used industrially in many ways, from the pigmentation of paints to the hardening of other metals. The radioactive form of cobalt is produced synthetically from natural cobalt and is known as cobalt-60. Cobalt-60 is produced when normal cobalt particles are placed in a device in which they can be bombarded with neutrons. This bombardment is done in a cobalt machine, and it is this instrument which the patient sees when he enters the treatment room. The massiveness of the treatment machine comes primarily from the amount of lead shielding required to protect both worker and patient from an overdose. There are a great many forms of this machine. In cancer treatment by cobalt-60 the cobalt machine makes it possible for the cobalt-60 to give off powerful gamma rays. These gamma rays can be meticulously directed to any spot on the body. Gamma rays are powerful and deadly, but can be life-giving when used against cancerous conditions.

By means of the very precise management of the cobalt machine the radiotherapist can direct radiation at any place, in varying amounts, for any given length of time. Of course the amount of radioactive exposure that the body can tolerate is severely limited, and there is a point at which excessive radiation works against the patient. This was the shortcoming of early forms of radiation treatment. For this reason, as powerful and useful as cobalt-60 is, it has its limitations and restrictions. No part of the body is inaccessible to the cobalt machine, but not all tissues of the body can be safely irradiated. The amount of cobalt-60 given a patient is measured in rads. One may receive a very mild dosage measured in the low hundreds of rads, or 10,000 rads, or more. Dosage at this magnitude is generally used only in advanced or extreme cases.

Cesium-137, the electron beam, and supervoltage are additional forms of treatment in the field of radiation, each of them using either a different source of radioactive material or dispensing their element in a different way. These additional tools in the storehouse of radiotherapy are available for special situations or as additional support in general treatment by radiation. Radioisotopes are radiation-charged elements that are sometimes placed in the bloodstream or tissue either as metals or as liquids. Radioactive gold, although not as useful today as formerly, is still an element used in the field of radioisotopes.

Irradiation as a form of cancer treatment continues to occupy a fundamental place in our treatment of the disease. New forms of this treatment, new instruments, and additional elements all help to provide continued faith in irradiation as a major weapon in the fight against cancer. These forms, instruments, and elements, as well as the technicians who administer them, are available to any person with cancer. They constitute one of our major sources of hope when cancer comes.

The third major field of cancer treatment is that of

chemotherapy. This is the science of placing in the body
certain chemicals that act to eliminate or control the
cancer that is present. It is the most experimental and
undoubtedly the fastest changing of the three major
categories of cancer treatment. Nearly every day some
new chemical compound or new synthesis of present
compounds is produced that will eventually find a place
in the fight against cancer. There are so many chemotherapy drugs today that one would not be able to list even
a fraction of them here. There are literally hundreds of
them. I will include a few of the names at this point
only because they are some of the most commonly used
ones and might very well be familiar to many who have
had chemotherapy treatment. Methotrexate has long
been a basic tool in the fight against leukemia and other
forms of cancer. Daunorubicin is a useful drug in produc-
ing remission in acute lymphatic leukemia. Daunomyvin
is another leukemic weapon, especially with children.
Vincristine, prednisone, vinblastine sulfate, mustine,
thiotepa, 5-fluorouracil, stilbestrol, and 17-hydroxypro-
gesterone caproate are just the beginning of an almost
endless list of chemotherapy compounds presently
available or in use by the chemotherapist.

These drugs are administered in one of several ways,
but the most common technique is that of intravenous
injection. The Fenwall Pressure Bag has recently sup-
planted the gravity drip system in the use of many of
these drugs, since it permits the patient to be mobile while
the drug is being administered. Other methods of ad-
ministering chemotherapy elements are orally (tablets or
capsules), by needle injection, and by incising the flesh
for placement of the element. A great part of the research being done today in the treatment of cancer is

being done in the field of chemotherapy as science looks more and more to chemistry for assistance.

There is an additional form of cancer treatment which may or may not be considered a fourth category: the field of immunology. It is new and still very experimental, but more and more effort is being directed to its development. Immunology is the approach to cancer treatment having to do with triggering into action the natural immunity factors in the human body. Science is quite convinced that, just as we can now immunize persons against diphtheria, smallpox, or rabies, it is only a matter of time until we will be able to immunize persons against cancer. This would mean a greater understanding of the natural immunity factors and processes of the human body than we now have, and the development of means by which those immunity factors can be activated. Yet immunology is an exciting possibility for eventual control of cancer and it may prove to be the most lasting and effective control of all. A major effort is going on now in laboratories and research centers to increase our knowledge of the entire science of immunology. At the present time there has been nothing like a cure or vaccine or serum from work being done in the field of immunology, but we can continue to be hopeful that such might eventually be. Perhaps the most dramatic disclosure of late comes from the U.S. Atomic Energy Commission in its report of the experimental use of BCG (bacillus calmetteguerin). BCG itself is a strain of tuberculosis bacteria used for many years in anti-TB vaccines. In May of 1972, Dr. Edmund Klein of Roswell Park Memorial Institute in Buffalo, New York, reported that he had successfully treated with BCG immunotherapy five advanced cases of breast cancer in human beings.

The five cases, he said, were all in varying degrees of remission or states of arrest.

So great is the interest in the possibilities of BCG that a ten-nation conference of scientists was held in October, 1972, in New York, to discuss its use and further development. BCG is but one of several new and very experimental drugs now being researched or applied in the treatment of cancer.

As exciting as this field of immunology is, all workers involved in it caution against expecting too much from it too soon. Immunology is just one of many avenues being pursued in man's long fight against cancer. We must not be too surprised, however, if immunology finally proves to be the basic method of controlling cancer. If this does prove to be true, it will mean that we will have learned more about the human body than we now know and more about the antitoxin systems contained in that body. But science is convinced that, just as we can now immunize the human body against many other dread diseases, someday it will be possible to immunize against cancer. In the light of man's increasing knowledge and skill it should come as no surprise if the prediction proves to be true.

In closing this section on prevention and treatment of cancer I think it is necessary for us to understand that the medical approach to cancer treatment involves the use of not just one, but sometimes two or three, of these major categories of treatment. Surgery is often followed by irradiation of the affected area. Radiation treatment of an infected part may not be adequate in itself, and in that case the physician will advise surgery. Chemotherapy may be administered after both surgery and radiation. This is to say, then, that while we still die of cancer in great numbers because we still lack basic knowledge about cancer, it is also true that we continue to live in great numbers after having had cancer. This is possible to an increasing degree because we have available to us the wide and diverse resources of surgery, irradiation, and chemotherapy to make sustained life possible. When the forces of immunology are added to that system of resources it is plain that as severe and killing as cancer may be, we are miles forward in our treatment of it and our eventual mastery over it.

Chapter 5

WE RESPOND TO CANCER

BECAUSE WE ARE ALL such "human" human beings, subject to the stresses and feelings that are a part of being alive in the world, we know with certainty that the onset of any dread disease, emotional upheaval, or sudden crisis brings about within us a surge of responses and reactions to those experiences. There is never any question about our reacting. There is only the question as to how we will react and how we will handle our reactions as they arise. Cancer is one of life's experiences that draws forth deep and sometimes life-changing response. There is so much dread associated with cancer; it brings upon us so many thoughts of death's prospects, thoughts of the dramatic and sometimes permanent changes it can effect, that we cannot avoid being caught up in the grip of profound feelings.

In this chapter we will discuss some of our responses. Those discussed here are by no means the only ones we encounter. They are simply representative of the wide range of reactions we make to critical experiences. Each person makes his own response. That response, or series of responses, will be determined by his particular situation. Depending upon how much preparation we have had for the confirmed diagnosis of cancer, depending on the prognosis, the location, and what the treatment is to be, we may experience one or all of the responses described here or others not described. Often these responses come, not one at a time, but all in a rush. We move from one response to another in hurried succession without being at all aware of the responses we are making. Things are too rushed and confused, and the responses are too automatic, for us always to think rationally about what is happening.

From my own experience with cancer, both in loved ones and in the wide range of persons who have been a part of my ministry, I have learned rather clearly, I think, that cancer is such a traumatic event in our lives that in the beginning we must depend more upon intuition and native strength than upon any rational thought process to see us through. I want to share three kinds of responses with you in the knowledge that at least a good part of those who read this book will be acquainted firsthand with what I am saying. I know that my experience is not your experience. In a very profound way each cancer sufferer has his own experience and his own set of responses to the coming of cancer. There is a common understanding in this Family that we do not lay bare secret things. I do wish to record here, however, what I believe to be a universal set of responses to the cancer situation. Our adjustment to that situation is a part of the response we make and whatever the response may be in any individual case, we can be assured that we are one with a host of others who have felt as we now feel. That is one of the joys of belonging to a family.

SHOCK

I found many years ago that the first and most predictable response we make to the news about cancer is

that of shock. The word "cancer" has such a fatal con-
notation, and it conjures up so many unknown anxieties
and perils in our minds, that shock probably remains our
most commonly shared response within the Cancer
Family. In medical terms, "shock" is described as "a
state of circulatory collapse, frequently associated with
insufficient return of blood to the heart, and manifested
by persistent deficiency of blood flow to the peripheral
tissues." [8] What this means in everyday terms is that
the diagnosis of cancer, the realization that cancer has
come, acts so powerfully upon our bodily system that
parts of that system lose their ability to function normally. Quite a number of writers in the field of cancer
treatment indicate that shock is almost always felt to
some degree by the cancer patient and by his loved ones.
"We found a tumor," is sometimes the way the news is
brought. "We had to do a radical mastectomy," is another common way in which we learn the extent of our
malignancy. There are other forms for the coming of the
news about cancer. Those of you who read this book will
know the variety of those forms. I have heard many
such words spoken to many patients and their families:

"We could not get it all."
"There was nothing we could do."
"I am afraid we have bad news for you.
The cancer has spread to the lymph glands."
"Your daughter has six months to live,
perhaps a little longer."

How many times have we heard those words, or others
like them. We remember how we felt and how we re-
acted. Perhaps the most common initial form of shock is
that which drains our strength and will from us. There
comes over us in those first moments after learning about

the presence of cancer a rush of inward emptiness. We can feel an almost physical draining out of our strength, the coming of a weakness that makes us go limp, makes us feel the need to sit down or lean on someone for support. Sometimes a feeling of indescribable sadness comes, with that surge of weakened will, or a feeling of enormous regret. Depending on the extent of the diagnosis by the physician, we may enter a period of time when we cease to think normally or logically, where we lose our bearings, our train of thought, and are confused mentally. I have known of families who had to be driven home from the hospital by a friend following the conference with the physician because the family members could not trust themselves to drive safely. How well I remember a young wife who was told, following surgery on her husband, that he had a very advanced and rapidly growing malignancy of the spine. So great was her grief and shock that she left the hospital, completely forgetting coat and rubbers, and walked out into a snowstorm coatless. Such is the extent of that initial experience of shock which comes upon us when the news is brought about cancer.

The full extent of shock's power is felt as time lengthens. Fortunately for many persons, shock is a reaction that is severe but that lasts for only a brief period of time. The return to normalcy comes soon and completely. This is the experience of perhaps a majority of persons who experience the response of shock. In other instances shock is more prolonged and has many manifestations. Sometimes we may begin to experience a lessening of our interest in daily work, in the household, or in our profession. Our relationships with people may begin to suffer badly as we lose interest in participating in those relationships, in holding up our end of the commitment required to make a relationship meaningful.

Things that have helped us in the past, activities that gave us excitement in life, and anticipated happenings or occasions may begin to lose their luster. Things, activities, and people that we have appreciated and looked forward to, and that have sustained us in past times, may lose their place in our scheme of interests and involvements. There often takes place a kind of disorientation, a losing of perspectives, regarding the real world around us. Many persons enter a period of prolonged sleeplessness, or insomnia. They walk the floor at night, or lie awake in the hospital, unable to find the necessary spirit of regeneration that comes with sleep. On other occasions, or in different persons, shock may result in severe experiences of sleep in which the person sleeps day and night in a kind of escape. He may become comatose. He loses contact with the world around him. Shock may cause us to experience difficulties with our breathing, with our normal pattern of bowel habits, with eating or reading or being entertained. Even in those situations where the diagnosis is clearly pointed toward complete recovery or cure, and where the recovery period is relatively brief, we may suffer a decrease in appetite, sexual drive or activity, and in interest span. Sometimes there is an obvious lessening of our efforts in showing appreciation, pleasure, happiness, thanksgiving, or contentment. In more severe experiences of shock we may endure periods of numbness, shaking, sweating, chilling, or weeping. There may be feelings of intense anger or resignation. At times we may experience lethargy bordering on paralysis. The vital signs of life may all be affected. If the cancer is deeply rooted or if the prognosis is poor and calls for extensive surgery and prolonged treatment, one or more of these symptoms of shock may be felt in unrelenting manner.

"Why are you cast down, O my soul, and why are you disquieted within me?" asked the writer of the Forty-second Psalm. This is an extremely human response to a moment in life's rhythm. The ancient man who spoke or wrote those words knew whereof he spoke. He reflects in this question a wondering about life and its fate, and his question is repeated over and over again in life today. The casting down of one's faith in the face of cancer, the disquieting and upsetting of the spirit in that moment of crisis, is a universal response. This disquieting opens to us enormous difficulties, but equally large opportunities. The disquieting of the spirit may be only another way of saying that we are moving toward that most destructive emotion of all, self-pity. The temptation to this is especially real if the prognosis is one that requires long-range treatment or radical surgery, or where the extent of the cancer brings one face-to-face with the possibility of death. So often a feeling of genuine helplessness sets in, a conviction that nothing can really be done, that life moves toward some inevitable end, that one has little to hope for or to contribute. Sometimes in that mood we put aside the willingness to fight for life, to use tooth and toenail in the struggle to hold back the ravages of the disease, to make a witness of courage or love while the struggle ensues. This is the disquieting of the spirit about which the ancient Hebrew philosopher wrote, and when he wrote it he spoke for all men everywhere who are troubled about life's adversities. This feeling, like anger or sweating or trembling, is an integral part of the emotion of shock. It does not come to all but I think it is safe to say that it comes to most sometime in the journey of facing and dealing with the fact of cancer.

Many times in my ministry I have seen cancer patients

with great possibility of full recovery become convinced in their minds that death was to be their fate.
Even when confronted with medical certainty about the
possibility of recovery, and even though surrounded by
the trusted word of family or pastor, there are many who
experience such a breaking of the spirit in those first
moments or days after cancer comes that they cannot
be swerved from the conviction that they are not being
told the truth. Patients have confessed to me frequently
that the doctors aren't really fooling them, that husbands or wives aren't as clever as they think they are,
that the conspiracy into which all those persons have
entered is seen very clearly by the patient. This disquieting of the spirit is a sometimes tragic thing to see
and it often takes time and effort and patience to overcome it, on the part of the patient and those who surround that patient with love and the richness of love's
healing.

I think this is a part of that disorientation of life of
which we have spoken. It is a kind of lessening of the
vital quality of perspective, the making of sure and
confident decisions. In those uncertain times of the spirit's
dismemberment the familiar gestures of love upon which
we have learned to depend may become unsteady, and
offers of present things and future affections are seen in
a lesser light. Turnley Walker, in his book on the experience of polio, has written: "The night has settled down
too thick for eyes to see."[9] That night is sometimes the
curtain of the disquieted spirit. We may not be able to
define it, or face it forthrightly, or even understand it, but
however uninvited it may be, however we may wish to
avoid or conquer it, it is a frequent visitor and a constant companion of cancer.

There is a second manifestation of shock that is commonly experienced among us when cancer comes, one which we call by that familiar old name, Panic. In many ways it is perhaps the antithesis of the despondency or the disquieted spirit of which we have spoken. Indeed the panic that sometimes comes upon us leaves no time or room for contemplation of our experience. Panic makes us want to do things in a rush, to accomplish a lifetime of things in a condensed period of time, to live and act at an accelerated rate of speed. Panic is, in a sense, a kind of flight from reality, and however human the response may be, it may also be an unrealistic and unnecessary response to cancer. There is no real reason why we should begin to rush around, stuffing a whole existence into a few days or weeks, being upset by the conviction that we must make decisions, give information, provide instruction, for those who are the center of our attention and concern. Mothers or fathers who come home from the hospital feeling that they must reorganize their entire household for the presence of cancer and its aftermath may very well be underscoring a lack of confidence in that family. If not this, then they may be taking from the lives of the members of that family the opportunity for responding in their own way to the cancer patient, a way that is finally more real and meaningful to them when it is found by them rather than provided for them. To say to husband or children, "From now on you will have to get along without me" may be saying, "From now on you may not know *how* to get along without me." I think this is in violation of the capabilities of most family members. Over the years I have seen the response of those husbands and children, wives and family members, and I know how quickly they come to the rescue, how they group together, share with one another, find meaning in taking on responsibility which they had not taken on, or been given, or perhaps even been allowed before. Instead of, "You won't have me to depend on much longer," how much more helpful and significant in the long run is it to say, "From now on I will learn to depend upon *you*."

A symbol of our panic about being away from our family for an extended period of time, or being taken away from that family by death, is that response on our part which makes us think we must reorganize everything in sight as quickly as possible. Usually we need do no such thing and I believe we may need to learn how to avoid this unnecessary response. I have known mothers of small children who set about frantically mending clothing, buying groceries, writing letters, and cleaning house as if there were to be no tomorrow for themselves or for their families. Almost without exception there are many tomorrows and we need at least to live at peace with those we have. I remember well a friend of mine, a colonel in the Air Force, who was diagnosed as having cancer of the larynx and could be treated, at least initially, with cobalt. This meant that his doctors were offering him a very special hope and that even if the cobalt failed to halt the spread of the malignancy, there was always the additional possibility of surgery. Yet this frantic man went for days without eating or sleeping. He spent hours in an attempt to overhaul completely the engine of a car he possessed when he knew little about mechanical matters. He painted part of his house (fortunately the back side), changed his will twice, called friends and relatives long distance with last-minute pieces of quite useless information. He became a worrisome neighbor and an upsetting member of his household all because he felt certain in his mind that he would either die immediately or live long enough to be speechless. The fact is that this man is alive and well today, having made a complete recovery from his malignancy, and is a successful practicing lawyer in his native state of Virginia. Today he looks back on those days of near-hysteria as a kind of unrelieved nightmare and he doesn't mind telling his story to others who face what he faced long ago.

Sometimes in panic we make mistakes. Even at best we may create situations or make decisions that we and others are called to live with, and from which we may suffer, for a long time to come. Sometimes in panic we say things which we live to regret afterward and which we can never quite recall. We may do hurting things to others, especially to those closest to us. We may become a difficult patient to deal with in our hyperactivity or our lethargy. We may quickly become impatient whereas our former self was patient. We may become insensitive to those who love us and minister to us and who feel their calling is to help us in every way possible. There are times when our panic causes us to be drained of the sound judgment and rational thinking that has characterized us previously and that we need rather desperately in the task of facing the necessities of the new situation of cancer.

I must add the reminder that there are times, when cancer comes, that we do indeed need to act quickly about one or many matters, to put things in order, to make preparations. There may be wills to make or change, fences to be mended, decisions to be made, conversations held, letters written, and a great many other things to be tended to. But I have found that there is almost always time to do these things unhurriedly and with proper planning, with an understanding of all the people involved and all the matters to be considered.

While I cannot suggest a foolproof method of fending off panic, I would say at this point that if we recognize that panic does come, and that it might very well be upon us now, or might come in a future moment of stress, we have taken an initial first step. Panic only adds to our disease and hinders the healing process. Given the rate of cancer cure, the remissions, the prolonged periods of time given us for treatment and recovery and adjustment, there is almost always no real reason why we should radically alter our tempo or rhythm of life. The changes will come, we adjust to those changes, and we are usually adequate to handle those changes. They ought to be allowed to come slowly, as they will, so that we can receive them patiently. Take your time! After all, time is on your side.

I would add another basic thought. Not everyone experiences shock in any conscious form, at least to the degree we have described here. Sometimes we have adequate warning and when cancer comes we are ready to meet it head on. It comes as no surprise and we incorporate it gradually into the pattern of existing life, or we change that existing pattern gradually. Also, what we feel of shock may be of very short duration, over and done with in a day or two, or a week at the most—if very quickly dealt with and replaced effectively with other responses of logic and thought and careful planning.

Yet, for all this, we know the wide extent of shock in the Cancer Family, and I am certain that many who read this book will know it firsthand as a constant companion. For this reason I find it important in my own life to understand it, to know its forms and symptoms, the available defenses against it, and how to wrestle with it when it comes. I also believe it is crucial that we understand that there is nothing "wrong" or shameful about these responses of despondency or panic. These are human emotions that arise in human beings, and doctors and clergymen and friends understand this. To an extent, shock is a necessary response in a variety of experiences. The human emotional system is capable of withstanding only so much stress, and when the intensity of the stress becomes greater than the system can handle, that system responds by shutting out the stress or blunting the stress by the forms we have just described. To receive more than one can bear in the emotional makeup of his body is to bring about the possibility of a far more disturbing response than just panic. Such stress, being more than the emotional system can handle adequately, may bring on collapse or a true emotional breakdown. Long-range mental disturbance may very well be the result. The function of shock is to regulate the amount or intensity of stress that is brought to bear upon the human emotional system. In automobiles we know this function centers around what we call the shock absorbers. I think that is an adequate comparison. If the human mechanism of shock were not available to us, we might indeed be called on to bear more than what is bearable, and we might give way before the onslaught. So what I am saying is that if one reacts to the coming of cancer in less than perfectly regulated ways, there may be a necessity for, and certainly an understanding of, the reactions that are made.

Yet in all this we continue to see the importance of growing beyond the depression or panic. One cannot remain forever in these states. Too much is at stake, too many decisions must be made, too much is apt to be

lost, for us to move too far beyond the previous equilibrium of life or the safe levels of response. The question
is, Can shock be helped? Can shock in any of its forms
be controlled, faced, and finally overcome? Or is shock
so automatic that it comes whether we will it or not and
remains as long as it will, regardless of any effort we
might make to dispel it? If there is no reason to believe
that one may rise above his depression or his panic and
to ask how it is all to be handled, then it is in order to
pose that question here. How do we remove this "night
too thick for eyes" from our spirits?

There is no question in my mind that persons possess
within themselves the capacity for this removal. This
certainty on my part comes from so many sources that I
can no longer have doubt that the possibilities exist for
such recovery. My life has been enriched by too many
experiences and case histories for doubt to linger. There
have been too many members of my own family afflicted,
and healed, for me to doubt this capacity. The record of
hospitals and churches and counseling centers is too long
and full of too many examples from real life for us to
doubt that the capability for recovery lies within reach
of each human being. There are too many great souls
of this earth who now live as witness to this recovery for
us to question either its reality or its possibility for us.
Unless shock is so severe and prolonged that it results
in genuine and debilitating emotional destruction, and
requires extended psychiatric care (and this happens
only in the rarest of instances), we may live our lives
today with the knowledge that there is built into our
psyches and personalities the resources that point us to
the regaining of stability and inner harmony. This never
should be taken to mean that one can always or neces-

sarily do all the recovering by himself, without some outside aid, but it does mean that one has the possibility
of acting, responding, and deciding, and this is his best
hope for the future.

I would say immediately that the first step in the recovery of one's equilibrium from either the pit of
despondency or the pinnacle of panic lies in the initiative of the individual. I will follow that by suggesting
that this is very likely the most difficult step, simply because it requires that one run counter to the very distress
that causes him to lack initiative. If initiative were all
there were to recovery, it might very well be that shock
would not occur in the first place. The truth is that few
people can look at themselves objectively and analyze a
condition while it is in the process of occurring. From a
hospital bed, however, from his home, or from the
security of his daily routine, he has a different view or
standpoint from which to take stock of his condition. In
that condition he recognizes that he may do one of two
things. By an act of will, by sheer determination, he may
resolve to go against his own inclination to despondency
or panic and react differently. This is a mental calculation
and it does not always result in immediate action, but it
is a necessary first step in the road toward new equilibrium. In that situation a person may need to force himself to do things that he does not want to do and that
he inwardly resists with all his might. He may need to
force himself to face people when his real desire is to
avoid people and withdraw. He will very likely find it
necessary to make decisions that he does not want to
make, simply because making the decisions helps him
toward a more rational understanding of what is happening to him. As much as possible one may need to con-

tinue, or to reestablish, familiar patterns of life which
have been disturbed or disrupted, with the knowledge
that these familiar patterns are necessary for sanity.

Across the years I have known a great many persons who have been immeasurably helped in this process
by a new effort toward religious faith. Sometimes in
crisis we fall into the mistake of expecting someone else
to provide us with our spiritual nourishment. There may
be, with the coming of cancer, a time when we are cut
off from the regular activities of our church or synagogue. Many persons feel this acutely. This does not
mean that one is not visited or remembered by the
members of those groups, but it does mean that one
cannot participate actively in those groups, and this
sometimes means the felt loss of an additional contact
with the world of persons. Yet this is the very time when
we may reexamine the meaning of our relationship with
those groups and the extent of our support of them.
Rather than waiting for the resources of the group to be
brought to us, rather than waiting for visits, cards, calls,
and assurances of support, we may make our hospital
room, or our space at home, the center of an outgoing
spirit. That hospital room or space at home might very
well become a kind of powerhouse, giving light and
encouragement to the surrounding community. We all
know, I think, that it is one thing to be cheered up and
supported, when we are sick, by someone who is well. It
is quite another thing, and quite possibly far more meaningful, to be supported and cheered by someone who
shares our illness or stress. This is in keeping with the
finest traditions of religious faith as well as the sheer
act of human living. I remember well a very great man
who, at the age of forty-three, went through an operation
that resulted in the loss of his right leg, his right arm,

and muscles in his right side. He was left partially paralyzed, able to be up in a wheelchair but not able to walk or work. This man has lived for more than twelve years following that series of surgical operations. He had formerly been owner and manager of a small printing firm and following his surgery he turned the press over to an assistant.

For a long time following his surgery this man lounged around home, felt useless, despaired of ever being a productive human being again, and generally felt helpless. Then, following a suggestion ·by a friend in the physical therapy section of the local hospital where he was going for treatment, this man went to work developing a unique service for persons involved in physical therapy activities in their homes. This service was geared especially for persons who were recuperating from a stroke, thrombosis, heart attack, or loss of limbs. His service consisted of preparing a series of cassette tapes which were made available at low cost to persons needing them in their homes. These tapes recorded the voice of our friend, who gave informal and newsy advice on how to do exercises, walk, learn to talk again after throat surgery, breathe properly, diet, gain weight, and sundry other things. The tapes were made available through the physical therapy department of the hospital or directly from this man. He makes no money at it since the tapes are prepared and distributed at cost, but he has fulfilled a desire to be of help to others, and since the tapes record his own experiences they are especially meaningful to others who use them.

Whatever may be our particular difficulty or need, I believe we may rise above it in significant ways by taking a first step, making a decision that points us in the direction of new purpose and meaning for life. If we do not do this for ourselves, it may become increasingly difficult for any person to do it for us or to help us to any extent.

We must not forget, however, that our own resources are not the only ones we have when cancer comes. There are times when we cannot in fact help ourselves and in such times we are dependent upon the love and support of others at least to help us come to that point where we can do something for ourselves. We are surrounded, when cancer comes, with persons who love us, who want to help us, who are concerned for us, and who in most cases have some degree of power or capacity to nourish us in our experience. This is true regardless of whether we live in the midst of a loving family, in a nursing home far from our children, or isolated in some place alone in the world. We are never away from people who would come to minister to us if they knew of our need. Every community has within it groups of people related to churches, social service agencies, community volunteer groups, and professional bodies which are organized to do this kind of ministering. However alone we may feel, or cut off from the mainstream of life, the fact is that we are not alone. The expression of need is the way to call these resources into our lives. Within the family we see this healing fellowship in its most dramatic form. Husbands and wives are closest to this healing method in the deepest way. By ministering to each other, they provide the warmth and encouragement and spirit of caring that is crucial to recovery or even existence itself. Our physician is a primary source of support. Even though he may be without an overwhelming bedside manner personality, he is here to advise, support, and even comfort. Our family clergyman, minister, priest, or rabbi is sometimes a neglected part of this healing process. I am always saddened by this because religion and healing have always been, and are now, united in their purposes for human life. Friends and neighbors are nearly always close at hand and willing to enter into the experience of others. These persons do have the power to support and sustain us when our own power of self-support has become weakened. It remains for us to let these persons have a part in our lives in a new way. It requires a new appreciation sometimes for the effort of others, a willingness to let them come into the circle of our experience, and an openness to the understanding they can provide. The discovery of persons is a constantly recurring theme in times of crisis.

There is a third part of this healing process which moves us from the various results of shock. It lies in our understanding of the process of healing itself. I do know from experience that the more we know of the way in which healing occurs, the meaning of surgery, therapy, and treatment, the basics of bodily responses to medical treatment, and the intentions and methods of the attending physician, the more confident we usually are about the power of healing and recovery. For this reason I continue to encourage members of my congregation, and others about me, to read as much about the science of medicine as possible, to absorb through reading, conversation, television, and other means, a store of knowledge about diagnosis, treatment, and surgery in the field of cancer as well as other diseases of human beings. Just the gaining of knowledge itself, a new awareness of the rapidly growing science of medicine, is a tremendous source of encouragement. A doctor, a librarian, a family

member, can provide these resources for you if you need
help from them. It remains to the bearer of cancer to
take advantage of what there is.

Finally, one will never neglect the ministry of the
medical profession itself in times of sickness. When we
begin to count up the resources that can move us beyond
those manifestations of shock we recognize that the ways
of an enlightened medical science stand near the top.
Available to every patient with cancer today is a carefully selected and prescribed series of steps. These steps
may be related to the cancer itself, as a part of the
treatment, or they may be related only to that experience of shock that accompanies the cancer. The physician has within his reach a selection of drugs that are tried
and true. These drugs can provide a lift from depression
and a lessening of panic. The doctor knows what to
prescribe and how to prescribe it. These wonder drugs
are often only temporary expedients, and both the doctor
and patient understand this, but they are a part of the
healing process just as much as surgery or cobalt therapy.
In addition to this the doctor may provide other means
for meeting effectively the stress and anxiety of our cancer experience. He will be able to assist us in gaining
new strength and inward resolution. Good communication between patient and doctor provides this and it is
available for all.

In all these ways we see how we are surrounded by
forms of healing and help. In fact, we are almost overwhelmed by the enormity of them. There is no reason
today for any person to suffer needlessly from pain, depression, or panic. However severe shock may be,
whether it is just temporary or of a longer duration, there
is help available. We must learn to use this help. This

"night too thick for eyes" can be lifted with the coming of the morning of healing. We must learn how to welcome this healing.

FEAR

"No one ever told me that grief felt so like fear. I am not afraid, but the sensation is like being afraid. The same fluttering in the stomach, the same restlessness, the yawning. I keep on swallowing." This is the way C. S. Lewis describes both fear and grief in his little book *A Grief Observed*.[10] In these words I think Lewis speaks for most of us in touching on the fear that is so real and ever present when we live with the reality of cancer. Whether the fear we have is about ourselves, whether it is carried on behalf of some loved one, or felt in our concern for a friend or neighbor, it can be a gripping, swallowing kind of fear which is mighty hard to dispel.

This fear is born of a real situation of course. It comes out of our knowledge that cancer is present, that it poses grave problems, that it is a crippling, pain-producing, sometimes killing disease. Who can be immune from fear produced by that sort of condition? Our fear is real when it is rooted in the knowledge that a benign tumor may become malignant, that a clean bill of health today guarantees no good health tomorrow, that successful surgery once performed carries no certainty of continued cure. How many times have I been present in waiting rooms of hospitals in anticipation of that moment when the surgeon comes to tell the family the results of his work on their loved one. How many times have I heard the words, "We found a tumor," or "He has cancer." In those moments fear is like a rumble of thunder or flash of brilliant lightning across the room. It bangs on the walls and tips the lamps and echoes across the room. It is hard and bitter and real. Whatever may be the assurances of the surgeon that the surgery was successful or that the tumor was benign or that there is nothing to fear, the patient and family fear anyway, and all the words of assurance that there is no need for fear do not erase it. It has a tremendously strong staying power. It is natural and human, and one should never be ashamed of it, nor be hesitant to express that fear or share it with family, friend, pastor, or surgeon.

Now fear is always a natural response to cancer, in some degree or other, but it is important to know that not all fear is necessary. It is also important to know that it can be dealt with creatively. Just as we have antidotes for other forms of affliction of mind and body, so there are available to us certain important medicines for fear. The reason for suggesting this is that while fear is sometimes a necessary response to crisis, putting us on our guard against something that threatens us and permitting us to prepare for battle, fear can sometimes be destructive. It can work against our self-interest, it can retard our healing and recovery, and it can sometimes be a barrier to the efforts of others to minister to us in healing ways. For this reason I believe it is helpful for us to learn something about how and why the fear comes and how we may prepare ourselves to face it. To remain a clear-headed, functioning, performing person in the midst of our cancer experience is one of the requirements leading to successful handling of the cancer crisis. If fear takes over too completely, one ceases to be an asset to himself or to others and in fact one becomes a liability to both.

What is it we fear when we say we are afraid of cancer? Is it the cancer? Yes, but in a far lesser degree than we suppose. Sometimes what we really fear is the feeling about possible death. We freely confess that death stalks the cancer patient and wherever the cancer patient goes death goes too. We want to live as long as we can in this world. Death is something we have natural fear about and there is no question that its possibility haunts us when cancer comes. Shakespeare's Hamlet spoke of this in the famous soliloquy which proclaims that the very mystery of death's meaning makes us want to avoid it. Hamlet meditated:

> Who would fardels bear,
> To grunt and sweat under a weary life,
> But that the dread of something after death,
> The undiscover'd country from whose bourn
> No traveler returns, puzzles the will,
> And makes us rather bear those ills we have,
> Than fly to others that we know not of?

Whatever else Hamlet might have been, he was certainly a man with great insight into the uncertainty of death's estate.

For all this I have come more and more to the conviction that death is not really what we fear most when we think we fear death. Evidence for this conviction comes to us from a great many sources as well as from personal experience with death and dying. In a very pointed statement about this fact Dr. Charles W. Wahl, associate professor of psychiatry, University of California School of Medicine, Los Angeles, has written:

When we fear death intensely and unremittingly, we fear instead, often, some of the unconscious irrational symbolic equivalences of death. Hence, the fear of death is in reality two things: a realistic concern that some day we shall cease to be and, secondly, a variety of other anxieties which parade under the panoply of the death fear, and these are varied in character and scope.[11]

Such insights as this point me to a conviction that when cancer comes it is not death we fear so much as life. Any fear of death is preceded by questions having to do with the interim period when we still live. When the presence of cancer is confirmed the questions come all in a rush, mostly unconsciously and automatically. "What will I do now?" "What will become of us?" "Will there be enough money?" "What will the children do?" "Will I be able to stand the pain?" "Will my husband still love me?" "Will I still be a woman?" "Will I still be a man?" These are questions having to do with life, not death, and they are real and poignant. The truth is that it is life which provides us with uncertainty, anxiety, and fear and it is in the midst of life that these questions must be wrestled with and these anxieties faced.

One of the regrettable things about these questions and anxieties is that they are almost never as severe or difficult to solve as we initially think they will be. Almost without exception things are handled by the patient and the patient's family in such a way that problems are solved and the anxieties thus lessened. While there is almost always an initial time of confusion and mistake-making, the long-term picture is almost always one of things getting done decently and in good order. In other words, much of what we fear about life is really a fear of ghosts that never materialize. I remember something that D. H. Lawrence says in his poem "The Ship of Death":

The flood subsides, and the body, like a worn sea-shell emerges strange and lovely.

And the little ship wings home, faltering and lapsing
on the pink flood,
and the frail soul steps out, into the house again
filling the heart with peace.[12]

Let us dispel some ghosts, then, and recapture the re-
newal of life that Lawrence speaks about here. I am
certain in my own mind that one of the greatest helps in
facing either death or life lies in knowing exactly what we
have when we have cancer, what we face for the future,
and how we may deal with it. My experience has been
that the lessening of anxieties sometimes hinges on the
strengthening of information. Many persons continue to
be afraid of cancer to such an extent that they will not
ask for information about it and about themselves, and
even refuse this information and explanation when it is
provided. One day while I was typing away at this page
in the book, in preparing the manuscript, a person asked
to read what I was typing. In reading the sentence just
before the preceding one, that person said: "You can
count me with those who don't want to know anything.
If I had cancer I wouldn't want anybody to tell me anything because I wouldn't want to know what I had or
what it would do to me!" Similarly, there is many a
person who goes for ten years without an examination of
her breasts or who puts Campho-Phenique on a sore in
the mouth that hasn't healed for six months. Day by day
persons suffer needless mental anguish because they will
not ask their doctors for information or explanation and
really aren't listening when those doctors come to explain. Physicians have no particular wish to press information upon patients who have no wish to receive that
information and many doctors proceed cautiously when
it comes time to do the explaining. I would add, of

course, that sometimes doctors could be far more profi-
cient in this than they are, and that they could do more
than they do to overcome the information gap that often
exists between patient and doctor. Yet we do know that
when information about cancer, its origins, prognosis,
and treatment, is honestly shared by the doctor with the
patient, when that information is shared between patient
and family or between patient and pastor, there is an
enormous release of anxiety and tension, and of the
ever-present fear. I will add that physicians, for the most
part, are more than willing to take the time to explain,
describe, and instruct throughout their entire relationship
with the patient. It is a wise patient who will say to his
doctor, "Doctor, tell me about cancer." To do this is to
take a mighty step forward in gaining freedom from fear.

The book *I Remain Unvanquished,* by Alice and A.
Dudley Ward, is a true account of Mrs. Ward's battle
with cancer. She speaks of the fear about cancer that she
met among sales clerks when they were asked to help fit
her for underclothing after her mastectomy. A mastectomy normally leaves a harsh scar running across the
breast area of a woman and sometimes, depending on the
extent of the surgery, scars that reach under the arm,
across the neck, and through the general shoulder area.
Mrs. Ward tells of the natural reluctance of saleswomen
to help other women in the fitting of the specially designed brassieres for women after mastectomy. She says:

My disfigurement revealed a dimension of fear in people
that I had not noticed before. How many women live in
constant fear that this may happen to them! I discovered
this in the dressing rooms of fine stores as sales clerks
would gasp and suddenly leave as they saw the scars
and burns. I soon learned to ask for the head sales person
when I went into the department. I would explain to her

that I had had a mastectomy and required certain types of clothes, and that I needed a mature saleslady whom my surgery would not upset. So I learned not only to protect them against shock, but also to protect myself against unpleasantness.[13]

This is a statement about fear of life from living persons, not fear of death from dying persons. And it shows us graphically that only as we see, examine, discuss, analyze, and talk through the experience of our cancer with persons who know how to listen and advise will we really overcome that most fundamental fear of all, the fear of life.

A second step in the dissipating of our fear is the development of lines of communication with loved ones. We have already touched on the *need* for this communication. What I am saying here has to do with the *depth,* or *degree,* of that communication. The word I want to use here to characterize this kind of communication is *honesty.* For a husband and wife to say to one another, "Now don't worry, everything will be O.K." is one thing, and sometimes it may be the right thing. It is quite another thing, and a necessary one, for husband and wife to come to that point where they can say, "Do you think my surgery will make any difference in our marriage?" or, "Let's see if we can make some decisions about the future." This is the honest approach to cancer, whether the condition is one requiring short-term or long-term treatment, whether the prognosis is good or not good. Every day in homes and hospital rooms there is a drama played out in this dimension of dishonesty. Certainly we know that there are times when it is required that information be withheld from a patient or from a family member. This is true when the patient is still in a critical condition, or perhaps when the patient or family member is aged. Each family must determine what decisions must be made in these situations. Of course the physician can always be of help in such times. But beyond this there is everywhere in the experience of cancer a needless addition of anxiety because patient or family will not ask for, exchange, or receive information and advice that could help to relieve the anxiety and accompanying fear.

"She doesn't know she has cancer" is one of the symbols of this. These words of instruction are given to pastors, friends, and others—yes, even to doctors—as those persons make themselves available for counsel and support. The meaning is clear. The patient does not know she has cancer and we do not intend for her to know. I wonder how often they ask themselves whether or not the patient might *like* to know. I will share a secret with you. I think the patient knows! That feeling is a product of countless experiences with patients and their families caught in the panorama of the cancer drama. The conspiracy of silence may be carefully structured and carefully guarded. But I have looked at too many patients who "didn't know" with the feeling that they knew very well. In those times of conspiracy, who really is it that spares the other, the family or the patient? I believe that very often the patient does know. There is something too basically intuitive about the human personality, and we know too much about cancer, its symptoms and its effects, for a patient not to have at least suspicions about this disease. Unfortunately the patient often consents to this conspiracy, indeed even originates it, pretending for the sake of not hurting someone or thinking to avoid needless grief. On the whole it does not work out well.

What is left out when this conspiracy of silence is allowed to develop and continue, what is omitted from the experience, is communication vital to the healing process. This process has to do not only with restoration to physical health but with the healing that must come to the spirit and the mind. There is no doubt that honest sharing of experiences of fear, doubt, the threat of death, the threat of the future and the present, contribute immensely to the store of sustaining strength available to both patient and family in the presence of cancer. This honest form of communicating the entire range of cancer-related concerns enables one to examine his own life and thoughts more deeply, to enter into new and unexplored depths of personal relationships with loved ones, and to look ahead in a far more confident way than ever before. The stage for this kind of honest sharing of concerns and anxieties and fears is set for us by the very nature of the cancer experience. Unless the cancer involved is only a minor irritation, easily and completely erased, the presence of and treatment for cancer is the kind of experience that normally causes us to want to talk about things. It often prompts us, certainly enables us, to share deeply in ways never before explored or experienced. We continue to observe the fact that the cancer experience creates a new readiness on the part of most persons for a discovery of the important. It is the kind of experience that prompts us to set aside the trivial, the momentary, the easily discarded things about life, for a new attempt to discover, or rediscover, what is important and lasting.

"Let's talk about it now" can be the beginning of this deepened discovery of our own selves and our relationships with loved ones. Dr. William Menninger of the Menninger Clinic in Topeka, Kansas, once said that the failure to "talk it out" was a basic omission in the healing process. The Bible adds a new dimension to this when it says, "Perfect love casts out fear." Perfect love means loving others enough to be honest with them, rather than thinking our love for them gives us an excuse for being dishonest with them. We discover that love is always strong enough to weather the cancer crisis and its possibilities, and to move us on toward deeper knowledge of ourselves and of our relationships.

There are many other forms of fear, of course. There are other remedies. The man of religious faith will turn easily to the resources and disciplines of his faith for the facing of fear. I think we begin to face that fear when we begin to look closely at the reasons for the fear, and it is then that we discover that fear is based more on what we do not know than on what we do know. The rest follows. This includes the will to live, a determination to see things through, a realignment of life, if this is required by the situation, a new awareness of the way in which love grows when fear is cast out. "Nothing in life is to be feared. It is only to be understood," said Marie Curie, a victim, due to radiation, of cancer, the very disease that her discoveries eventually helped to treat. That insight has stood a great many persons in good stead over the years. I believe it is a profound lesson for us in these moments of our encounter with the disease that took her life and that sometimes takes our lives, or threatens to take them.

For the cancer patient and his family, who must face the fear related to cancer, the starting point for release from that fear is an understanding of what it is we face and what we must now do to survive. In that understanding I believe there is release from the fear. If not release, then certainly there is a strengthened ability to handle the fear and to face it more adequately. This may be our creative response to fear.

Hope

"Hope is grief's best music," says an old Spanish proverb. I happen to like the saying because it gives one a very profound insight into another important response we make to the coming of cancer. We have spoken so far of the response of shock and the response of fear, and of the ways in which we might meet these responses advantageously. Now it is time for us to remember that beyond the shock and above the fear, after the withdrawal and in the midst of the panic and the dread, there looms the possibility of another response, one that is at once conscious and unconscious, controllable and uncontrollable. It sometimes accompanies the first two responses, often tends to mitigate the severity of their presence, and almost always outlives and overcomes the first two. I refer of course to the response of hope.

The longer I live as a participant in, and observer of, the goings-on in the Cancer Family, the more I am overwhelmed by the hope that pervades and persists in and through the experiences of my fellow human beings. This is all the more remarkable when we remember that we are dealing with a disease that is surrounded by so much hopelessness. It is often called a hopeless disease. The proverb quoted at the beginning of this section is a necessary reminder, I think, that grief is always with us in our Family. It is born in the center of our experience of pain. It comes with the threat of death, is present during those periods of prolonged absence from our families and homes while we are patients in the hospital, and is a by-product of all those anxieties which press in upon us whether we are a patient or a loved one of a patient. Hope is always the companion of grief. There are times when grief is borne outwardly, in the tears of which we need never be ashamed (who has not cried just thinking about the suffering of a loved one?) and in the words we speak in order to convey our feelings. It is borne inwardly as well and manifests itself by our feelings of sadness, the gestures we make, the movements we initiate toward others. These expressions of our grief are generally useful tools in the releasing of anxiety or the sharing of distress with another.

This comes home to us in a real way when we see how this grief is made bearable by our hope. Somehow these two emotions of human life go together like Gilbert and Sullivan. How well we know in this Family that the greatest degree of suffering often gives birth to the strongest degree of hope. None of us understands this as fully as we might, but I see the workings of it and I stand in awe of its possibility. "Hope springs eternal in the human breast" is more than poetic musing. It is a real fact of our existence and is another way of saying that hope is an indestructible element in the human predicament. I believe this response of hope is a part of the adjustment we make to cancer. I do know that hope influences these responses and humanizes them, as well as makes them possible.

Therefore in all our experience with cancer we should learn to value more highly, and to use and cultivate more effectively, our capacity for hope. I say this because there is a surprising amount of despair around the wards and clinics and patients' bedrooms these days. I am not sure but that some doctors add to this despair. To tell a patient that he has six months to live, or that his cancer is inoperable, or that no further treatment is possible for him, without reminding him that life does not consist in length of days or that there is compensation of things given for things taken away, is to deny the role of the doctor as healer. Oh, I know that the physician might well insist that he is a physician and not a philosopher. But I accept no such claim! A healer is a philosopher and a theologian and a humanitarian or he is not a healer! The physician may have a degree in medicine and he may be a practiced surgeon and he may be considered an expert in his field. But if he cannot speak a word of hope, if he cannot in fact lift up the hope that does indeed exist within the experience of the human spirit, if he cannot say something regarding the meaning of the experience of suffering, then he will remain only a practitioner of his art, which in reality calls him to be a healer of the human spirit as well as a healer of the body. It should be pointed out that physicians are careful not to provide false hope or to lead a patient into an erroneous sense of confidence, and they are well advised to do just this. But the physician may often offer to the patient a word of encouragement that is more powerful than his surgery, or a quality of character from his own life that is more lasting than his chemotherapy. Which is to say of course that the physician, in the best sense of his profession, is a man of hope as well as a man of knife and suture.

In this day of enlightened medical science we see, more and more, that hope is not predicated entirely on whether or not a cancer patient is to live or die. Hope has a far deeper dimension than the physical life. I would say to anyone who has cancer, or to any member of a family where there is a cancer patient, that one of the greatest resources you possess in your battle with this disease is a hope that insists that life have *quality* in the midst of *quantity,* depth in the midst of length. Hope is that presence in every human life which insists upon the possibility of a victory of the human spirit even in the presence of the death of the human body. The annals of literature, music, religion, and the arts are filled with monuments created in remembrance of those who somehow touched the surrounding world with their hope in the midst of their suffering, if not their death. Michaelangelo in his *Pietà,* Joe Rosenthal in his great still life photograph of Marines raising the American flag on Iwo Jima, Tchaikovsky in his *1812 Overture,* and William Styron in his *The Confessions of Nat Turner,* all touched in a powerful way, or represented in a powerful way, the lives or experiences of persons who somehow surmounted the stifling and killing spirit of their surroundings to display their hope to an incredulous world.

Realistically, we know that cancer does threaten the hope we have about physical life, about the length or even the quality of it. A man who has lost his voice box and parts of his face to cancer can hardly be blamed if he questions his ability to function adequately in the world or to make a contribution to the community of persons. We know very well that cancer can take our lives. It may cripple us, cause us suffering that leaves telltale marks on body and spirit, take away our ability to enjoy life, handicap us in our effort to be productive, contributing human beings. This fact is best epitomized by the remark often heard after diagnosis has been made: "There is no hope." Sometimes in our inner spirits, in our survey of the future, in the prospect we have for things, we think this about ourselves or about those whom we love and for whom we suffer deeply.

Is there such a thing as a human being without hope? I have pondered this question for a long time. I have looked for the answer to it in hospital beds, in the literature of our time, in the many records left of those who have suffered, who have been tormented and persecuted, and who have died by the hundreds of thousands. In the end I have been drawn to a conclusion about it all. Yes, there are persons who are without hope, *if* we mean by that that such persons live *as if* there were no hope. Yet I have read the writings and autobiographies and chronicles of a lengthening line of sufferers, and I am convinced today that hope is everywhere present in the experiences of persons under every condition at every moment. Just as an example I would point out the haunting stories of Anne Frank, of Dietrich Bonhoeffer and Martin Niemöller, all victims of Nazi persecution, as evidence of the presence of hope in the midst of pure despair. Who can read the story of the plight of the Jews in the building of Israel after World War II, or the story of the Arabs displaced in that feat, or of the blacks living in South Africa today, without catching some of the feeling of hope that cannot be extinguished even, or especially, in the midst of horror and oppression. How deeply I believe in the presence and workings of hope in the worst of conditions, yes, even in the face and fact of death!

This hope is well founded. In fact, one of the greatest sources of hope for the cancer patient is in the picture of cancer research and treatment itself. After all, for goodness' sake, 218,000 Americans will be saved from death by cancer in 1974, and more than 2,000,000 Americans now living will eventually be classified as "cured." That represents an amazing compilation of hope in my estimation, for each person counted is a human being. The fact that the prevention rate and the "cured" rate both continue to move upward is heartening and glorious. One in three persons is now cured of cancer, and the American Cancer Society estimates that earlier cancer detection would make possible a large increase in the number

cured. Add to that the number of persons cured, or
healed, by new and improved methods of treatment, and
the figure may well become one in every two in a relatively short time. Who can despair in the midst of so
much hope?

The second ground of our hope is that found in the
prospects of cancer research. We do know that an increasing number of persons afflicted with cancer will be
cured with treatment methods and procedures now in use,
as those methods are improved. Many other persons will
be cured with procedures now only in the experimental
stage or yet to be discovered. This includes methods related to the three major categories of treatment: surgery,
radiotherapy, and chemotherapy. Even beyond that, we
know that many others will be protected from cancer in
the first place through preventive procedures. We have
previously touched on some of these preventive steps.
Today in universities, science centers, and the laboratories of private foundations and drug companies, research in cancer origins and treatment is a twenty-four-
hour, seven-days-per-week enterprise. While there is not
now available anything like a "cancer cure," no miracle
drug that will either *prevent* all cancers or *cure* all cancers, any drug anywhere that saves even one life is a
miracle of sorts, and these new drugs and treatment
procedures are becoming more and more available as a
product of the research going on around the world. Yes,
these new procedures and products will come too late for
many. They will come in time for many others. Some
of you who read this book will have your lives literally
saved by some new treatment or product. We must never
give up that part of our hope which is tied to new devel-
opments in cancer research.

There are many agencies and forces now working to

make this hope real and a part of the lives of an increasing number of persons. The United States Government has not always recognized the crucial nature of research for peacetime matters. It has spent billions of dollars for military weapons research and development over the past years and continues to spend enormous amounts of money on new weapons of destruction. It has never quite grasped the vision of such sums for health, education, welfare, and for the basic research required eventually to win out over cancer, arthritis, multiple sclerosis, and half a hundred other killing and crippling diseases. It has been estimated that had the United States Government put at the disposal of the medical and drug researchers the amount of money spent on missile research and development alone, many of the diseases mentioned above might have been conquered twenty years ago. This is not to say that money alone is the answer to disease research and treatment. Yet additional sums of money would have made it possible for more qualified scientists to remain in the research field, and it would have given them more tools to work with, more laboratories and equipment, and more access to one another and to conferences where information could have been exchanged and shared. Lacking these sums of money, many schools and research centers have had to make do with fewer staff members and with the lack of newer tools and equipment. Many groups concerned with research and treatment of cancer and other diseases have had to take to the streets in private fund drives for the money needed to carry on this work.

Slowly, but with an increasing sense of urgency, this is changing. In December 1971, for example, President Nixon signed the National Cancer Act, which provided 1.6 billion dollars for cancer research. The funds made available through the signing of this bill serve for the period 1972–1974. These funds are channeled into science centers and universities and laboratories where the basic research continues into our understanding of cancer. The American Cancer Society, as an independent agency, is one of our leading private forces in cancer research. In its fiscal year 1973 the American Cancer Society made 525 grants to 147 major institutions in this country and to scientists working both in the United States and abroad. The total amount of money approved for these grants was $25,652,737. Such an amount of money is pitifully small when compared to the enormity of the problem and to the number of grants applied for but turned down because of lack of funds. Yet, taken together, these amounts, coupled with other independent funding agencies and the United States Government, together with many universities and drug agencies, provide a tremendously hopeful picture of future research in the field of cancer. The American Association for Cancer Research, Southern Research Institute, Kettering-Meyer Laboratories, National Cancer Institute, and Sloan-Kettering Institute for Cancer Research are but a few of the institutional names associated with research in the field of cancer. Howard Temin, David Baltimore, Sol Spegelman, Jeffrey Scholom, and Melvin Calvin are just a few of the doctors, scientists, and technicians who have increased our knowledge of the entire range of viruses, DNA, RNA, immunology, and cell structure in the whole field of cancer research.

One of the things the National Cancer Act of 1971 did was to authorize the creation of fifteen new Cancer Centers as well as to provide additional assistance for those centers now in existence. These Cancer Centers are seen by medical science as a gigantic step forward in man's fight against cancer. Speaking before the Conference on Planning Cancer Centers held in Washington, D.C., on December 9–10, 1971, Lane W. Adams, executive vice-president of the American Cancer Society, said this about the proposed new Cancer Centers:

> The Cancer Center appears to be the ideal combination of the features essential to cancer research: the collaboration between the clinician and the research scientist, the collaboration of the many bio-medical disciplines; the availability of the latest technologic developments, and the opportunity to concentrate on targeted clinical problems and to solve them through teamed basic and clinical research.[14]

What these Cancer Centers will do in fact is to provide a central clearinghouse for the entire work of education, research, treatment, and service in the battle against cancer. These centers will serve as a kind of "Pentagon" for cancer control in the future.

The time will come of course, is perhaps even close at hand now, when major new discoveries will be made in research and treatment of cancer beyond what is presently available. When that time comes we know we will pay homage to the hundreds of workers and agencies that labored so long and arduously to bring about new hope for cancer cure. The fact that this research is now moving ahead with such feverish pace is one of our finest symbols of hope in our fight against cancer.

There is no way to speak of hope in these matters without touching on the hope offered by religious faith. Hope forms such an integral part of most religious ties, and it is so deeply rooted in the doctrines and beliefs of religious traditions, that to overlook the hope made available in religious faith would be extremely shortsighted.

Nearly all the great religions of the world point their adherents toward a way of life superior to that known by their nonbelieving neighbors. This "superior way of life" is defined in any number of ways. Sometimes it is an offer having to do with the rewards and quality of life discovered in this life for the here and now. Sometimes it is an offer of some better way of life in a world to come. This superior way of life has to do with the manner of life lived by the adherents of that religion, with qualities of courage, faith, love, or perfection of character. To the unbeliever, and even perhaps to some men of faith, much of this is somehow unrelated to what one believes to be deeper meanings about life and human existence. Yet by these values and doctrines, by these promises and standards, civilizations have been built and have endured, individual persons have been lifted out of destructive or nonproductive patterns of life and pointed to more creative patterns, and the tones of entire cultures and civilizations have been touched and perfected by those values and systems. Christianity is one of the examples of this "more perfect way" as Paul the apostle described it in I Cor., ch. 12. The "more perfect way" is not the sole property of Christianity, however. The faith of the modern-day Hebrew, a faith continued through centuries of persecution, dispersion, and cultural assimilation, remains a faith of great and abiding ethical power.

This is to say that within religious faith there is a real and conscious hope that in the midst of man's ordeal in his life, in the midst of his pain, anguish, torment, and failure, there is still open to him the option of rising above his predicament to a new life of courage and victory. Religious faith is rooted in commitment to a divine power, be that God, Allah, Jehovah, or Ahura Mazda.

Faith thus is related to the ability of that divine power to sustain persons, to bring about change and improvement, to be the means by which healing is made possible, and the welfare of other persons promoted. As Dr. Karl Menninger writes in *Man Against Himself,* "Religion has been the world's psychiatrist throughout the centuries."[15]

I speak here as a Christian, and while I do not know the full extent of the mysteries of the faith to which I belong, I do know from my commitment to that faith that it provides enormous support for the healing process in persons. Christians believe in a God who is actively involved in the care of souls. They put their trust in the man Jesus Christ who is called the Great Physician. Christians believe, with good evidence it seems to me, that this religious tradition does provide the stimulus for the highest form of physical, emotional, spiritual, and social health. As to whether God provides this healing power directly through his divine intervention, whether Christ becomes the healer on his own initiative or on the initiative of the believer, whether the cleansing and healing power of the Holy Spirit is given on condition or given freely, Christians are not always in agreement. Why healing and continued good health is given to one person and not to another, withheld or given without apparent reason, is not at all clear at this time. Perhaps it will become more clear in time. Why the righteous suffer and the ungodly prosper is an additional perplexity, a situation that seems unfair somehow to our concepts of fair play. Yet, perhaps this is not as complex as we sometimes think. The Christian God is not a god who plays hide-and-seek with persons, a benevolent divinity who dispenses rewards for goodness and withholds those rewards when we do wrong. The Christian Scripture provides the key to our understanding of this process when it says: "He makes his sun rise on the evil and on the good, and sends rain on the just and on the unjust" (Matt. 5:45). That is to say, the power of religious therapy and support is dependent not on a capricious god but on the capabilities of persons to understand, appropriate, and assimilate that therapy.

This is the excitement found in today's new thrust for a more complete union of insights from both religion and science. Today, as never before in the history of civilization, there is a merging of the concerns and powers of the objective data of medical science and the truths of religious faith. The direction of this is toward a holistic approach to the human person. This is stated most succinctly in a paragraph from a small booklet called *The Healing Church*. This booklet summarizes the Tübingen Consultation held in 1964 under the cooperative auspices of the World Council of Churches and the Commission on World Mission of the Lutheran World Federation. This confederation was made up of a small gathering of individuals, mostly physicians. In the closing meditation of the booklet, Charles Germany writes:

> We know that the healing of bodies apart from life in (Christian) fellowship is as incomplete as launching ships in dry harbours, or sowing seeds on stony soil. On the other hand, when healing does take place in the setting of the corporate life, or if it can involve ingrafting into the body of Christ, then healing has truly and wonderfully taken place because one abides in him who alone is the source of health.[16]

What is being said here is that the healing of bodies takes place only in the larger dimension of life and thus always involves the lives and experiences and support of others. It is precisely at this point that science and religion begin to act mutually in support of the person, be he sick or well. Science and religion are never in conflict with one another except in the limited minds of some scientists and believers who see nothing of the deeper meaning of the holistic ministry of their vocations. In its best sense, healing on any level, stimulated by any source, administered by any agent, is a blending of all the powers and all the resources available to men today from both science and faith. Men such as Russell Dicks, William and Karl Menninger, Wayne Oates, Paul Tournier, Seward Hiltner, Erich Fromm, and Rollo May pioneered in bringing about such a synthesis of medicine and religion. They were met eagerly by scientists who had been waiting long for such an overture. Most of these men from both religion and science provided a significant step forward in our move toward a holistic ministry of healing. Today in schools of medicine and schools of theology, students, physicians, scientists, clergymen, and philosophers gather together to draw from one another the insights available for a more effective and coordinated theology of healing. In all of this, religion plays its foundational role of providing the atmosphere, the reasoning, the motivation, and the concern for persons through which total healing may be made available to the patient. In terms of the daily life of the patient this means that through the counsel of clergymen adequately trained in the best tradition of the healing ministry, through the discipline of one's own faith, through participation in the life of healthfully motivated faith groups, one has every reason to believe that healing can be gained, that it can remain, and that it will sustain him through his future days. This is a wonderful hope and how foolish we are to neglect it in those times when we, or others, have such need of it. Cancer is one of those times.

There is a fourth avenue of hope in which I believe we discover a dimension of experience which has power to influence and enhance these other sources of hope previously mentioned. I would refer to this as the frontier of the human spirit. The cancer patient is a pioneer of sorts, since he charts a course of action and response. This charting of a direction involves decisions about both the present and the future. For that patient there are few if any landmarks. For that person the experience of cancer is new and unfamiliar and not all the counsel and advice and previous experience of others is adequate for his facing of the experience. That is not to say that there are no landmarks or that others have not left some signs along the way for the later traveler on this road. The history of human life has a large record of cancer history, and the sufferers of that disease have left an impressive record of their feelings, decisions, victories, despondencies, and growth. What we are saying is simply that none of these experiences can really guide the present cancer patient too well. No one else's pain alleviates our pain. No other cure guarantees our cure. Not another's victory over the disease makes us any more sure of our eventual victory over the disease. Each of us must come to these experiences of pain, cure, and questioning by his own path, beating down the dense brush, clearing away the obstacles, making a path toward the future.

Many years ago a writer by the name of John Howard Griffin wrote a tremendous little book called *Black Like Me*. This was the story of Griffin's adventure, as a white man, into the world of black life. This book was a kind of "first" in showing the white world what a black man faces in our predominantly white society. It was a book about incredible depths of prejudice and hate di-

rected by whites toward blacks every day in our society.
John Howard Griffin has written an article called "The
Terrain of Physical Pain" in which he says:

"In the realm of the spirit it is not so much what we do
as what we allow to be done to us," Gerald Vann once
wrote. Certainly, at the deepest levels of human creativity,
a part of genius has been the ability of men to allow
themselves to be used as a sort of filter for experience;
to accept the experience imposed on them without even
judging its value, allowing it to enter, allowing it to teach,
and then letting it come out in some form of expression—
prayer, silence, music, contemplation, art.[17]

What does Griffin mean by that? Essentially I take it to
mean that there is a freedom open to us in determining
not only what cancer will do to us but also what we will
do with cancer. What will be our response to it now that
it has come? Will we let it antagonize us, embitter us,
make us less than our former selves, separate us from
former friends, alienate us from family members, interfere with the commitments we have made to values?
Shall we let cancer turn us into an "outworn shell by
life's unresting sea," inert and unresponsive to the ebb
and flow of life's joys? This may indeed happen to us, for
there are many who permit it to happen to them. Yet
there is something else we can do, and that "something
else" is precisely our hope. That "something else" is our
privilege in choosing the weapons of combat, choosing
the time, the place, and the manner in which we will do
battle with the adversary. We may deliberately and consciously war against cancer in a way chosen by ourselves. That is a privilege offered us by life. We are not
able to choose the treatment, the degree of the malignancy, the time given for surgery, recovery, or continued therapy. Those ingredients of our battle are set for

us pretty much by others. Our freedom in choosing weapons and strategy lies in our uses of the spirit, which we have previously spoken about. Since man is a spiritual being, he possesses an indomitable power to engage cancer with that spirit. We are indeed filters for the experience of cancer. We may collect the daily residuals of that experience as if these residuals were afflictions, a collection of curses, or a monstrous injustice done us by something or someone, or by nothing in particular. Having collected these in our minds, we may rail against them, throw bitter resentments into the wind, show hostility to the surroundings in which these experiences take place. Indignities done to our bodies by cancer, or by those who treat us for that cancer, the reflections and reactions of well-intentioned but sometimes thoughtless friends, the hurt and pity shown by family members, the true suffering of the pain within us, the dulling of the bright senses by all manner of drugs meant to help us, are the residuals which we may collect and retain and let fester to the detriment of our spirits.

Or we may do something quite different from that. We may filter and retain a different set of experiences and feelings, discovering them to the benefit of ourselves and others around us. The good done to us by a great host of people, the moments of joy in the midst of sadness, a new insight gained somewhere along the way, the appreciation felt for something given or learned or experienced, mastery accomplished over some temptation to self-pity or bitterness, a contribution made by ourselves to the astonishment of friends and family, the feeling of God's good presence in moments of quietness or need, are the things that we may retain and enlarge upon in the dimensions of the human spirit in the experience of cancer.

Who can deny that this is possible? Too many witnesses have left their record of mighty victory gained for us to lack assurance that light shines in darkness, that one can be stronger than his weakness, that the "hopelessly ill" or "terminal" patient can provide words and an example which will cause others to take heart, that life can be affirmed in the presence of death. Alan Paton helps us with this when he writes: "If my suspicion is true, then I vote for the universe we have, where we have our joy that has been made real by our suffering, as the silence of the night is made real by the sounds of the night. And we have our suffering too, made real by our joy." [18]

Well then, the question is not really about whether or not we may have hope. It is really a question of what the scope of our hope will be, what we shall do with the hope we now have and with the hope that shall be gained tomorrow. It is not so much a matter of what becomes of us as it is a matter of what we shall become, through cancer. We may decide that, my friend. In a sense probably, we are *required* to decide that as a member of the Family. That decision involves faith, appreciation, response, will, and gutsy fortitude. It involves an enormous amount of questioning sometimes, but also an enormous amount of affirming. Remember the words from one of the prayers of Michel Quoist:

> Thank you, Lord, thank you.
> Why me, why did you choose me?
> Joy, joy, tears of joy.[19]

This affirming of life in the midst of death's threat is a sometimes severely fought contest and the issue remains in doubt for many who read this book. That question has to do not only with the threat to the body but also

with threats against the spirit. But let there be no hesitation in living as a hopeful person, for we do not *become*
a hopeful person so much as we *live* the hopeful person
we already are, or are prepared to be. Albert Camus,
who knew so much of life and death, gave us all a great
boost in the spirit when he wrote:

> One may long, as I do, for a gentler flame, a respite, a
> pause for musing. But perhaps there is no other peace
> for the artist than what he finds in the hour of combat.
> "Every wall is a door," Emerson correctly said. Let us
> not look for the door, and the way out, anywhere but in
> the wall against which we are living. Instead, let us seek
> the respite where it is—in the very thick of the battle.
> For in my opinion, and this is where I shall close, it is
> there. Great ideas, it has been said, come into the world
> as gently as doves. Perhaps then, if we listen attentively,
> we shall hear, amid the uproar of empires and nations,
> a faint flutter of wings, the gentle stirring of life and
> hope. Some will say that this hope lies in a nation; others
> in a man. I believe rather that it is awakened, revived,
> nourished by millions of solitary individuals whose deeds
> and works every day negate frontiers and the crudest
> implications of history. As a result, there shines forth
> fleetingly the ever threatened truth that each and every
> man, on the foundation of his own sufferings and joy,
> builds for all.[20]

That is hope!

Chapter 6

CAN RELIGION HELP?

THE QUESTION POSED by this chapter heading is a perennial one among people everywhere. In a sense I suppose it is unanswerable, yet of course it is answered every day. Much of our discussion here must of necessity deal with allied questions such as what we mean by "help," and help for whom, and under what conditions. Do we imply here that religion can always cure cancer, take away pain, give full confidence, make one completely adequate for the experience of suffering? We must say immediately that no such thing is implied. Such an assumption would run counter to what we know of both religion and suffering, and counter to much of our human experience. Do we mean to imply on the other hand that religious faith does have healing properties, that it does provide immense resources of strength and endurance, that it enables us to incorporate suffering into our daily lives with a confidence of bearing that suffering, that it gives us assurance and even undergirdings of joy? Yes, we do mean to imply that plainly. What we say here about the relationship between religious faith and any experience of suffering is a product of what many have known and experienced in their own lives, and of the evidence that comes to us daily from the world of medical science. In this chapter we will attempt to show the difference between religion as a false promise and religion as a personal, unifying power. Our evidence is simply human experience. It is this experience which permits a housewife to say:

> This experience began an involvement that would remain with me the rest of my life. I realized that I had to learn the meaning of this psalm [23] in a wider, deeper, and higher dimension. In the moment of my greatest aloneness, the Spirit taught me the twenty-third psalm. I knew at that time, and have reinforced my knowledge in later years, that God does not fear cancer. God is greater than cancer. He holds the ultimate victory. By daily relating to his presence, I, too, can know victory.[21]

Likewise, a man untrained in religious matters can pose a question about why God permits suffering and receive this reply:

> According with my whole position, I say that God is active here. The age of miracles is still present with us and I will not presume to set a limit in my belief as to what God may do. Therefore, I look for him on every hand; I look for tomorrow with great expectation! Faith in God is this very expectation and the prayer of faith is not simply a breath upon our lips, a weak voice lost in the clatter and roar of the real events of the world; it is itself an event and the means of creative alliance with him.[22]

What is being said here is that religion does help those within the Cancer Family. I do not ask you to accept that on my word alone. I want to offer you something from my own experience, but from the experiences of others as well. I must confess there is no way for me to be completely objective about this. Religious faith has played too great a part in my own life for me to view it completely objectively. I have seen too much healing, too many persons brought into new relationships with God and themselves, too much victory gained over adversity, too much profound joy in faith, for me to be always objective. Yet I believe my convictions at this point are based on real life experiences and can be tested by time and the witness of others, and for this reason I do not hesitate in the least to share those convictions here. I believe they are shared by a great many others.

One day not so long ago I was in Chicago waiting for the airport limousine to pick me up from my room at the airport motel for the next part of my flight to Miami. It had been a wearisome but necessary trip and I was anxious to get it over with, to be back home with my family, and to begin making some use of what I had gathered as a result of my trip. The room I occupied in the motel faced out on a long dense thicket hedge that was an obvious natural haven for birds, rabbits, mice, and sundry other species of wildlife. One could see nests back in the thicket that generations of birds had probably used, and there were paths cleared through the underbrush that told of the sojourns of other creatures in that urban jungle of growth. I must confess I was surprised to see so much wildlife in that congested and noisy part of the city. The motel is wondrously convenient to the airport, but it is constantly under attack by planes coming and going at every hour of the day and night. How wildlife can survive that dense concentration of noise I do not really know, and I guess I am surprised that human beings also can stand it. Be that as it may, I was standing in front of the rear window of my motel room idly watching the thicket while the television added noise to the already noise-saturated atmosphere. While I was standing there, my attention was caught for some reason by a brown bird that kept flying to and fro in the thicket. Since the bird did not fly beyond that particular area of the thicket I kept my eye on it and began to catch a kind of pattern to its flight. I discovered that the thicket had a section in it where the tops of the branches were heavily matted together by dense vines and leaves. Inside that pocket was a kind of special protection from the outside world. Covered by the dense thicket hanging overhead and protected from the front by the crisscrossing of branches, the pocket was a hiding place and shelter from the congestion of the environment. I do not know much about the hearing system or the nervous system of birds, but in watching that brown creature I was convinced that the flight of the airplanes every three minutes or so caused the bird great anxiety. Whether that affected the bird at the point of its hearing or whether the vibration or sight of the planes affected something else in the nervous system of the bird I cannot say. I do know that just as regularly as the planes left the runway or came down onto the runway the brown bird flew into the pocket and remained there for a minute or two, then flew out again in the two minutes of relative quietness. On schedule, without exception, it entered the pocket again and again with the departure or arrival of a plane. That pattern of the brown bird's activity was so automatic that I am sure it had been carrying it out for a long time. It seemed to me then, and it seems to me now when I think about it, that that pocket of dense thicket provided a place where the noise of the planes was muted and a respite was provided from the surrounding stress. The bird had obviously intended to stand its ground and not forsake its place in the thicket. That was its home. It was just that it needed a place where it could escape from the severity of the noise or the sights and somehow be reassured. I saw clearly that the bird was not afraid to come out of the thicket following the arrival and departure of the planes. In truth, that frail little bird was able to reenter the noisy world because it had time to recuperate and reorient itself during its time in the thicket.

Cancer, like all other disease or hurts of the human body, brings to us a dis-ease of the human spirit. We have already written of the responses we make to the coming of cancer. We know that the presence of this dis-ease brings anxiety and uncertainty to each person, and to each person's family caught up in the experience. In the light of this anxiety and uncertainty we reach out automatically for whatever supports, encourages, helps, heals, and comforts us. This support, encouragement, and comfort is absolutely crucial to our experience and without it we live in isolation and loneliness. In any time of need we depend on something or someone to sustain us. This is not weakness or illusion or self-deception. It is a very basic need, and we must appreciate the person who is strong enough to recognize his need and to obtain help for himself for that need. If it were otherwise, we would never go to a doctor, have our clothes cleaned, take a bath, talk to a friend, seek out a marriage counselor, have our car fixed, or look for any other kind of help in our inability to do adequately all those things for ourselves.

When cancer comes, there is often a renewed interest in the power and therapy of religious faith. Our turn to religion is as natural and genuine as the flight of the brown bird to the thicket. I am convinced that this sensitive creature managed to survive in its hostile environment because of the recuperation of the thicket. Religious faith is recognized as a natural and genuine expression of the human spirit. That does not mean that it is recognized as such by everyone, of course. Some will deny the need for religion, for its promise or its hope. Indeed there are many today who believe strongly that any religion is a form of superstition and portrays human weakness. Denial of the creative and positive aspects of religious faith is well developed in our society today. Without doubt, religion has sometimes been an adverse influence on human good. It can still be this if the form of religion practiced is a denial of religion's inherent powers to free one from superstition, guilt, and selfishness. One must, I think, take into account the person, the past experience, the present situation, and the future conditions in determining what religious faith can do in any one case. We do know that religious convictions can work against the welfare of a person if those convictions, for example, lead him to neglect medical help in his disease. If one's religious experience and traditions have been limited to an environment where religious practices were oppressive, judgmental, negative, or burdensome, he may reject religious answers to his questions. If one has seen others live and die in expectation of a healing that did not come, he may reject not only the possibility of healing for himself but the source of that healing as well. If one has lived without faith, he may see a great inconsistency in asking for a state of faith now that he is in crisis. He may be content to trust medical science alone for whatever help can be given. These are decisions about life which we make every day in the family of man.

For all this there remains the conviction, held by enormous numbers of responsible persons in today's world, many of them without any particular commitment to faith, that spiritual assurance is a vital ingredient in the healing of the body and the mind. Religion that meets the highest qualifications of man's need for encouragement, love, self-respect, interpersonal relationships, and ultimate hope has proved itself of lasting value in the development of human life.

From man's earliest experience in the human situation, in good times and bad, he has called out for religious faith. As far back as Exodus in the Old Testament we discover the cry of anguish of persons in travail: "And the people of Israel groaned under their bondage, and cried out for help" (Ex. 2:23). From their experience of deprivation and distress these Hebrews spoke a word born of surety when they affirmed: "And God knew their condition" (Ex. 2:25). These Hebrews spoke the conviction of generations of persons since, that God does indeed know our condition and that he enters into that condition with power and release.

We are reminded at this point that throughout the long, tormented history of the Jewish people this conviction of God's identification with human suffering and need was lifted up time and time again. "As the Lord lives, who has redeemed my life out of every adversity . . ." was the way David affirmed the divine solace. When the tragedy of his newborn child's death overwhelmed him with grief, David "arose from the earth, and washed, and anointed himself, and changed his clothes; and he went into the house of the LORD, and worshiped" (II Sam. 12:20). What we see here is the inexorable pull of the human being in adversity to a source of hope and deliverance, and his response to that source for the deliverance given. In dark times of distress how strong this pull is, how seemingly natural it is, how adequate it proves to be, in bringing us closer to the wellsprings of life. And when it came time for David to put off this mantle of his earthly sojourn, he drew upon that vast reservoir of faith to proclaim: "For who is God, but the LORD? And who is a rock, except our God? This God is my strong refuge, and has made my way safe" (II Sam. 22:32–33).

Our recognition of the relationship between religious faith and well-being, our discovery of the power of religious faith to sustain and support us, is perhaps nowhere better described than in that soaring drama we call the Book of Job. This ancient record reveals to us the most human description possible of our response to pain and adversity. In and through Job we are brought face-to-face with the pure meaning of suffering, and the relationship of that suffering to our inner crisis and our felt need. The circumstances of Job's life bear repeating. A man of great wealth, esteemed in his community, an elder among his people, possessor of influence and power, blessed with a large family, surrounded by great lands and spacious herds of livestock, secure in the condition of his daily life, Job appears to us as a true sheikh of old, benevolent and generous. We see no cloud upon the horizon of his life, no wind to sweep over his domain to trouble the waters of his serenity. Then, without warning, tragedy descends, and this tragedy is so immense and so persistent that we are left awestruck that Job survives at all. The great herds of cattle and camels, his flocks of sheep and goats, are all taken away by marauding bandits. Job is left without that most normative possession of Oriental times, his livestock. Then, the news comes to him that all his servants have been slain in the fields. No sooner has this tragedy been revealed to him than he is notified that all his children, his sons and his daughters, "the fairest daughters in all the land," have been buried in death under the fallen timbers of their house. There are few parallels in all of literature, or of human life, to such an enormous calamity.

The Book of Job is an ancient literary drama, composed for, and produced on, the stage. It is not hard for us to imagine the excitement and controversy that was raised among the theatergoers who witnessed this drama of human and divine activity. The fact of its dramatic form and composition does not at all lessen its power as a statement of what men do in suffering, how they respond to that suffering, how they are weakened or strengthened in that suffering, how they bless God or curse God in those times. As calamities descend one by one upon Job, he maintains his dignity and his faith. "Naked I came from my mother's womb," he says, "and naked shall I return." (Job 1:21.) Yet not even then was life through with its affliction for Job. Soon this steadfast man is covered from head to foot with an excruciating physical affliction. In pain that must have been almost beyond enduring, Job begins that process of accommodation and discovery which comes to each of us in times of adversity and which we cannot avoid when cancer comes. There may be times when we, like Job, are tempted to bypass our spiritual resources. Job was tested at this point: "Let the day perish wherein I was born," he laments (Job 3:3). He considers the possibility that God himself is the cause of his suffering: "For the arrows of the Almighty are in me" (Job 6:4). He longs for death as release: "I would not live for ever. Let me alone, for my days are a breath" (Job 7:16). Job thinks of his affliction as being the result of his sin: "I have sinned. . . . Why hast thou set me as a mark against thee, so that I am a burden to myself?" (Job 7:20.) Job seeks forgiveness as a way of release: "Why dost thou not pardon my transgression and take away my iniquity?" (Job 7:21.) In these questions and declarations, so reflective of our present searchings, Job begins that process of reaching out for some communion with religious faith: "O that I knew where I might find him!" (Job 23:3.)

Who of us cannot identify with that searching? How often have we turned inward to faith and outward to God through what we say, what we pray, what we confess to one another and to ourselves in the privacy of thought? How much the literary Job shares our real-life experience of the search for faith!

But shall we leave Job here without an answer to his question, without some hope, or promise of hope? Shall we leave him to doubt, without strength to lighten his load or faith to guide him into his uncertain future? No, for everywhere in this great drama the assurance comes through as bright rays of light through the tree-tops of a dark forest. It finally remains for the young man Elihu, young in years but wise in faith, to share with Job the key to the understanding of faith. In line upon line, Elihu lays bare the nature of God:

> It is the spirit in a man, the breath of the Almighty, that makes him understand. (Job 32:8.)

> For his eyes are upon the ways of a man, and he sees all his steps. (Job 34:21.)

> Surely God does not hear an empty cry, nor does the Almighty regard it. (Job 35:13.)

> He also allured you out of distress into a broad place where there was no cramping, and what was set on your table was full of fatness. (Job 36:16.)

When Job contemplates the wisdom of Elihu and recounts his own past experience and the insights gained from his distress, he affirms: "I had heard of thee by the hearing of the ear, but now my eye sees thee" (Job 42:4). This statement of faith's assurance has been repeated again and again by those who have discovered the resources of God. Through those resources strength was gained, power recovered, inner conflict resolved, and peace established with others.

Job is not alone in his capacity to see the hand of God in human adversity. Nor is he alone in his ability to permit that presence to do its work of healing and comfort. Psalms, a rich storehouse of response to human travail, and of human achievement in that travail, speaks for all of us with this note of awareness: "O God, thou art my God, I seek thee, my soul thirsts for thee; my flesh faints for thee, as in a dry and weary land where no water is. So I have looked upon thee in the sanctuary, beholding thy power and glory. Because thy steadfast love is better than life, my lips will praise thee. So I will bless thee as long as I live; I will lift up my hands and call on thy name" (Ps. 63:1–4).

That call is answered throughout the psalms. "He who dwells in the shelter of the Most High . . . will say to the LORD, 'My refuge and my fortress,' " affirms Ps. 91. The meaning here is not so much that we avoid the human predicament through faith as it is that this human predicament becomes bearable through spiritual resources. The psalms speak of the condition and distress and deliverance of all of us when they reveal the plight of men who wander in desert places of the spirit: "Some wandered in desert wastes, finding no way to a city to dwell in; hungry and thirsty, their soul fainted within them" (Ps. 107:4–5). The deliverance: "They cried to the LORD in their trouble . . .; he led them by a straight way, till they reached a city to dwell in" (Ps. 107:6–7). The response of joy: "Let them thank the LORD for his steadfast love" (Ps. 107:8).

There is no end to this record. In a time of immense change, when the individual seemed to have lost his place in the midst of enormous distress in the nation, the prophet Isaiah recaptured the concern of God for persons in his great sermon on divine love:

> Have you not known? Have you not heard? The LORD is the everlasting God, the Creator of the ends of the earth. He does not faint or grow weary, his understanding is unsearchable. He gives power to the faint, and to him who has no might he increases strength. Even youths shall faint and be weary, and young men shall fall exhausted; but they who wait for the LORD shall renew their strength, they shall mount up with wings like eagles, they shall run and not be weary, they shall walk and not faint. (Isa. 40:28–31.)

How deep and powerful is this expression of human confidence in the healing work of a healing God.

It remained for the Christian faith to bring into clearest focus the true nature of God as one who entered fully into human experience. In the Christian faith we see clearly this power for which men seek in their relationship with God. We see man's joy and gratitude and deepened capacity for trust. Jesus is often referred to as the Great Physician. We see clearly how this was manifested in New Testament times. Page after page of the New Testament records the extent of God's healing through Jesus Christ. Jesus healed leprosy (Matt. 8:1–3), blindness (Matt. 9:27–29), emotional distress (Mark 7:24–30), epilepsy (Mark 9:14–27), demon possession (Luke 8:26–33), arthritis (Luke 13:10–14), and fever (John 4:46–51). It was said that Jesus "went about all the cities and villages, teaching in their synagogues and preaching the gospel of the kingdom, and healing every disease and every infirmity" (Matt. 9:35). In that sentence is the summation of the caring nature of God. That such caring, manifesting itself in varieties of ways, is physical healing, is hope, is strength gained through the presence of Christ beside our bed of pain, and is available in support of men and women who struggle to regain balance in life, is made clear in Jesus' teachings about the meaning of life, and is contained in the promise of Christ that we need never suffer alone. This multidimensional healing ministry, so rich and complete, ministering to the whole person, brought forth exclamations of joy, surprise, gratitude, and relief from those who surrounded Jesus. Jesus always conducted his ministry by carefully explaining that all his power came from the heavenly Father, and that all praise should be directed to the Father.

If the four New Testament books of Matthew, Mark, Luke, and John were the only record we had of the caring ministry of God, we might do well to be skeptical of its efficacy. But the whole of the New Testament supports the legitimate nature of this ministry. We know that the apostles maintained the healing ministry that Jesus established. In Acts, ch. 3, we are introduced to the later New Testament healing ministry. Long after Jesus and Paul had gone from the scene, James reminded the second-century Christians of the healing arts:

> Is any one among you suffering? Let him pray. Is any cheerful? Let him sing praise. Is any among you sick? Let him call for the elders of the church, and let them

pray over him, anointing him with oil in the name of
the Lord; and the prayer of faith will save the sick man,
and the Lord will raise him up. (James 5:13–15.)

Such a record of hope and courage gained, of support
received, of prayer answered, and of strength discovered
in the midst of trial cannot be taken lightly. It is the
conviction of men and women throughout the ages that
God is indeed "a very present help in trouble." On
that conviction hangs the promise of strength and new
life from our spiritual resources when cancer comes.

It is this conviction which gives us comfort and support today. To draw upon our spiritual resources is
natural and a daily experience for a great many persons. However we do this, whatever our need or our
response, we may be sure that we stand in a long line of
persons who have sought for, and found, the redeeming
power of religious faith.

Our turn toward faith then, as one of the many resources in the fight against cancer, is seen as a natural
and genuine expression of our needs. It is far more appropriate to confess that need than to deny it. That
confession may be manifested even though there has
been no previous commitment to faith. This, too, is a
natural step in our search for healing and wholeness and
strength. Nearly all religions speak of the availability of
religious nurture in times of crisis. For the person who
has lived by the power of faith, the onset of cancer
will almost certainly bring about a deepening attachment
to that faith. For the person who has not previously
lived by that commitment the discovery of religious resources may well be one of the most important discoveries made in that person's experience with life. In what we
know to be a natural confidence in faith's power a person
may find new and available strength and capability.

One's clergyman or spiritual adviser may be received in a new and more deeply appreciated light as he shares his experience and sympathy and counsel with the cancer sufferer. Friends and family surround one with words of hope and comfort which often come from their own religious intuitions. One's church or synagogue or house of worship may offer the support of a loving, genuine, enabling fellowship. A sufferer may find new interest in religious literature and in writings that tell of the experiences of others in similar situations. The bibliography at the end of this book will give suggestions for such reading. One may begin a more active participation in a religious fellowship as a means of finding new support and love. This is possible if the cancer sufferer is not confined, and it is always possible for the loved ones of the sufferer. The responses one makes to religious teachings, beliefs, and convictions are many and they are different for different persons. Yet it is my personal conviction that overwhelmingly, when the response is made, it results in new support and deepened trust.

Support for the view that religious faith is of genuine help in times of crisis comes from the medical profession itself. Dr. Raymond D. Pruitt, as chairman of the Department of Medicine at Baylor University College of Medicine, Houston, Texas, wrote:

Human illness traced back to its source in the individual patient almost inevitably provides a meeting place for the physician and the clergyman and a bright and challenging opportunity for the best efforts of both, one in support of the other. Communion between the ministry of healing and the ministry of faith is as old as man's search for God in the turmoil of lives beset by the malignancies of passions and plagues, of demons and death.[23]

Thus, in looking back over the long history of man's search for deeper meanings to life and experience one is struck with the tenacity and intensity with which he has held to religious faith. One is also struck by the extent of the benefits that have accrued to him in that search. It seems to me that there is ample evidence before us to suggest that this commitment to faith is a well-founded companion to commitment to all other values and forms and resources that elevate, sustain, and enhance the human family. The belief that there are available to us healing and correcting influences in human life is based on our understanding of man as a spiritual being. Man is always bones, hair, skin, and flesh, but he is infinitely more. Indeed, he is even more than intellect or thought or beholder of beauty. Man is spirit. He is one who has within him a force or power that enables him to endure sufferings as well as to contemplate the meaning of those sufferings. Man's existence is predicated on the basic truth that he is a spiritual being, or creature. This does not in any way deny his physical existence. It enhances that physical existence to a more elevated position. When the spirit is broken or even damaged, when the spiritual part of a person is denied or destroyed, he becomes little more than a grouping of bones, hair, skin, and flesh. "It is the spirit that gives life," said Jesus (John 6:63).

Scientifically we know the importance of this. How well the physician knows that the spirit is absolutely crucial to the recovery or continued well-being of the patient. A person may die of a spiritless condition just when the body is well enough to go on living. The physician surrounds the sick with influences that promote and enhance good health. Pleasant surroundings, cheerful staff (insofar as they can be cheerful), music through the intercom system, religious services through a chaplain, ready access to friends and family, a library of good reading material on wheels—all these are seen by the physician as aids, and necessary ones, to good recovery. These aids do not interact with a muscle, a bone, or a single, isolated organ. They interact with a whole person. They do not minister in any conscious way to a diseased leg or a broken pelvis. They minister to a living person, one who responds, feels, has emotions, is frightened or anxious; one who has willpower to be used and access to inner resources reinforced by religious faith. Dr. Paul Tournier summarized this well:

> Spiritual life involves the whole person, and not only the psychological processes studied by the psychologists. Dr. Maeder writes: "Faith is essentially the affair of the person." And Dr. A. Stocker: "It is the spiritual which makes the person." [24]

As for the brown bird in the thicket, there is for the human person a natural seeking after a place of refuge and healing in times of stress. The believer, the man of faith, will find this available when he turns to what he believes is the source and sustaining spirit of his life. By and large, the practicing believer will know how to do this. The man for whom faith is more difficult, the one who has not been previously close to the practices of faith, may be more hesitant or reluctant to take steps toward religious faith. He may be uncertain about the visits of a chaplain or clergyman. He may feel ill at ease with the advice of those who speak easily of religious things. He may act with restraint or even fear at offers of spiritual help or counsel. Men act in differing ways in those situations. In spite of all that, I am never far away from the conviction that new interest in religion is born of our need and that consideration of it may come much easier in times of difficulty than in times of tranquillity.

These resources for health, healing, and well-being are available to any person who reads this book. They are not the special property of any faith, any denomination, or any religious group. They are available because of the special nature of your own life, and may be brought closer to you by your clergyman, your hospital chaplain, or other religious adviser. They are available through the fellowship of your church, synagogue, or spiritual family. They are available in the privacy of your own home. They are available through the sacred scriptures of your faith, through prayer and contemplation. They are available through the disciplines of your faith and the sacraments. They are available when you need them and desire them. It does not matter much whether you are a practicing man of faith or previously of little faith or no faith. God does not keep accounts. He keeps no score of wrongs (I Cor. 13:5, New English Bible). He does keep watch over his children, and more especially when they suffer, it seems to me.

I believe in faith healing. This is not to say that I accept all the practices or claims of that discipline. There are, of course, a goodly number of charlatans and fakers in religion as in every other field. Yet we have always been aware of faith healing and of those who practiced that art. In times past, these "healers" were often found in tent meetings on vacant lots and in abandoned store buildings. Their services were characterized by religious fervor, evangelistic and emotional demands. We are well acquainted with the radio versions of these healing services. Later, some of them were presented on television. These healing services were sometimes filled with more heat than light, with loud and demanding prayers, wild claims of success and sometimes atrocious practices involving magic cloths, touch (the laying on of hands), and false promises. No one can really argue that under this intense emotional catharsis there were not some dramatic results, and that there are not people today who testify to complete physical healing as a result of these services.

Today, however, the art of faith healing is better grounded in the knowledge of both sickness and health. That is to say, the same basic insights that gave some legitimacy to early practices of faith healing have been brought to new and more valid stature. I accept wholly the belief that faith healing is a legitimate expression of the complete science of healing and wholeness. I cannot tell you how this form of healing really works. In fact, I have yet to meet a person with genuine healing powers who even tried to explain how it works. There is too much yet to be learned about faith healing for any person to be called an "expert." I do know that there are persons among us today who do possess "the gift of healing" and whose works of healing have been confirmed by scientific and medical authorities. The weight of evidence is too strong for the effectiveness of the discipline of faith healing for us to doubt its power. I am supported in this conviction by many who have studied this discipline thoroughly, and who provide authenticated evidence. Faith helps immensely in releasing us from fear, pain, anxiety, and guilt. Faith is a vital resource in filling us with a new sense of courage and meaning for life. To that extent there are many witnesses to the discipline of faith healing from the fields of science and medicine.[25]

Let me say a word about the actual practice of faith healing. In most instances this healing is practiced within a gathering of persons who are sensitive to persons and equipped to support the healing ministry in every way. These gatherings take place in surroundings that are conducive to the well-being of the petitioner. The traveling healing ministry of Kathryn Kuhlman is an example of such services. The quiet and restrained methods of Ambrose and Olga Worrall is another. It is my personal feeling that these persons, and others like them, do possess extraordinary powers of healing and that they conduct their services in the best tradition of faith healing. The Christian faith traces its beginnings to a healing fellowship and what we see today in healing services is a part of that tradition.

What I am saying here is that it is my belief that religious faith helps in maintaining healthful patterns of life, promotes good health during times of health, and provides support for healing during times of illness. Nothing in my faith takes me away from my own physician or denies the importance of medical care. At the same time nothing in my confidence in medical services takes away in the least from my belief that religious faith offers additional resources for health and healing beyond those possessed by medical science. I remember that great little saying on the inside front cover of *The Last Whole Earth Catalog*. That saying is: "The flow of energy through a system acts to organize that system." [26] I believe in this fundamental principle of the human organism and I am convinced that the energy released within the life of a human being through the power of faith promotes health and makes healing possible.

I believe religion helps. Whatever may be the condition of faith on the part of the reader, I will suggest that that condition be strengthened, renewed, or discovered, so that faith may minister to you in a deeper and more powerful way.

Jesus of Nazareth said, "I am the bread of life." That bread which sustains, fills, and nourishes us, and without which we cannot live as spiritual beings, is found in the healing acts and in the new life available to us after healing has come. It is provided through our religious faith day by day, generation after generation. I count on it. I believe you may too.

Chapter 7

DEATH

IN MARIA H. NAGY'S ARTICLE "The Child's View of Death" there is a description of several interviews held with children between the ages of three and ten regarding their conception of death. In one such interview one child reported his feelings in this way:

"Death does wrong."
"How does it do wrong?"
"Stabs you to death with a knife."
"What is death?"
"A man."
"What sort of man?"
"Death-man."
"How do you know?"
"I saw him."
"Where?"
"In the grass. I was gathering flowers."
"How did you recognize him?"
"I knew him."
"But how?"
"I was afraid of him."
"What did your mother say?"
"Let us go away from here. Death is here." [27]

Human beings die of cancer. That fact is real and inescapable. We have already stated that in 1974 approximately 355,000 persons will die of cancer in the United States, and that perhaps 3,500,000 will die of cancer in the 1970's. Many of these are persons who were cancerous and who could not be treated successfully. Some will be those who have previously reached the "cured" stage but are suffering a terminal recurrence of the disease. Many will be persons who were once free of the disease but who became cancer patients. Not all our advances in the science of research, diagnosis, and treatment will keep some of us alive after we have become cancer patients. For this reason I believe with all my heart that no book about cancer can ever be complete until it somehow touches on the fact of death and until it brings us face-to-face with the possibility and the meaning of death. As we see in the example just given of a child's attitudes about death, we are acquainted with death, we fear death, and we somehow wish to go away from the fact of death, if that is a possibility.

Death should not surprise us at all, since death is interwoven with life. In a sense we are born to die. Just as the presence of death in this interview, death is recognized as a kind of constant companion to living. During our lives we make the most of our time and opportunities, taking from life the pleasure and contentment and feeling of usefulness that are our right. All the while we know that life leads to the experience of dying. Sometimes we fear that fact, preferring not to think about it, discuss it, or prepare for it, and preferring to hide it in such terms as "passed away," "passed on," or "expired." At other times of course, in certain circumstances and for some persons, death is a welcome experience, ending what is often a burdensome or emptied way of life. All of

us live with the knowledge that death comes to all.
Until death takes possession of the physical part of us,
of course we fight it, scratch and scrounge around delay-
ing it, resisting tooth and nail the incursion of death
upon life, doing all we can to push death farther and
farther into the future. That effort may very well be
necessary and all to the good, since the human will, our
courage, our determination to live at all costs, is a crucial part of staying alive. All medical research and
treatment of the human body—and the mind, too—is
geared to pushing away death to some other time. Some
of the greatest recorded experiences of human life have
to do with the struggle to win out over death during a
particular time or experience. We will go on fighting
death and pushing it away because life is precious and
good and we want as much of it and from it for as long
as we can have it.

But we cannot do that forever. For a child with
leukemia, death may come at a tragically early age. A
brain tumor may strike the most outstanding young man
of college age. The young mother with a new child may
be a victim of cancer before her child can walk or talk.
Such is cancer, and such is the precarious nature of
human life. For this reason, given the nature of cancer
and its statistics, death is an ever-present reality in the
life of every person who has cancer anywhere in his
body. That fact leads us to seek the medical advice and
treatment that may save us for a ripe old age where we
finally die, not from cancer, but from some foolish ail-
ment like obesity or too much booze in the liver. But we
seek the prolongation of life because we believe that life
is of more value than death, and because for all the
unknowns of living we are willing to accept this rather
than the certain uncertainties of death.

Yet for all this, must we always look upon death as some kind of enemy? Is death always to be feared? I think not! We may speak of "dying before our time," but that is not quite right, as it seems to me. Who determines our "time" and who says our death is untimely? Have we not learned that the quality of life is sometimes more meaningful than the length of life, and that one may indeed live a lifetime in twenty years? Once I read something that I have long remembered, although I can no longer remember who wrote it. Whoever first stated these words uttered a profound piece of philosophy when he said: "While men must die there is open to them, nevertheless, the determination of how and in what name they are to experience death."

It is this insight into the experience of death and dying which means much to me as I ponder the death of so many friends and loved ones from cancer, and from other causes too, for that matter. The roll call of my loved ones taken in death grows so long that it threatens to outstrip the roll call of the living. In pondering this I am sometimes deeply impressed not only by the quality of life that characterized their living but by the strength of life that characterized their dying. I have known a great many persons who died in their teens, and many who died in their early twenties and thirties. These were young people, men and women, whose lives seemed to have come to some kind of fruitless end. Yet I have no difficulty in remembering that some of those persons (I think especially of a young high school girl) crowded what seemed to be a whole lifetime into a short existence in terms of years lived. I could tell you over and over again how many persons have confronted death from cancer with a great victory already won in their spirits.

The reality of death brings us face-to-face with things

that cause us to ponder deeply the meaning of life. I have witnessed reconciliation among family members, between husbands and wives, between parents and children, that might never have been accomplished through life alone. How many times have I seen persons let go of the transitory things of life in order to grasp new dimensions of beauty, faith, and love among the family of persons. I remember so well the young man in Dallas who, with both cancerous eyes removed, and with death only weeks away, holding up before his sightless eyes an array of books which he smelled, fondled, and leafed through, absorbing almost by osmosis of spirit the words and meanings of those books. I remember the twelve-year-old boy, his head swathed in bandages after removal of a brain tumor, his body immersed in ice water to hold down the soaring temperature, singing "Happy Birthday" under his breath to his brother, from a deep and fatal coma. The record is filled with victories won in the midst of death.

Men with strong religious beliefs may be sustained in the face of death by the promise of immortality. The conviction that life goes on in a different dimension is a great comfort when we think of having to leave behind an accumulation of love and life's achievement. Nearly all the world's great religions possess this hope of personal immortality. In the Christian faith this hope is based on the conviction that God is both creator and sustainer. Christianity holds that what God creates is good and that what he creates he sustains and conserves, including human life. There are many differences in what this may finally mean to individuals, of course. Whether this immortality is physical or spiritual, whether there is a consciousness of former existence, whether there is possibility of communication between the present

living and the past living, must all remain largely conjecture, since there is no universally acceptable way of
proving an answer one way or the other. It is, however,
the conviction of the Christian about God's nature, and
about his intentions toward his human family, that provides the hope of immortality held by that Christian.

Not all men share this conviction, of course. Others
see their immortality in a cultural heritage created and
left behind for others, a leaving behind of some achievement or example or gift which contributes to the welfare
of later arrivals. Some see their immortality genetically,
living on in the lives of the descendants of their union
in marriage with another. There are others for whom
immortality in any form or for any reason is quite without any meaning.

I for one see little cause for controversy in all this.
If there is immortality according to the conviction of the
Christian, then there is immortality, and no amount of
conjecture on our part will change that. If God wills an
eternity for those he creates, then he wills that for all
those he creates, not just for the privileged few. Any
other view, it seems to me, would bring us perilously
close to a capricious and even sectarian God. Such a
God would seem hardly capable of creating any kind
of immortality or of being a companion in that immortality.

The promise of something beyond this earthly life is
an important part of the facing of death for many
persons, but it is not the crucial point in my view. If we
live or die only to gain some future life, we may very well
have lived in vain and in denial of all we know of God or
of life itself. There is a deeper (and at the same time
higher) meaning to death. That meaning is found in the
reality of life. Only in life can we contemplate the mean-

ing of death. What is life for? How is it to be lived? What does it all mean anyway? These are the questions which give us our interpretation of death. Death but makes meaningful the gift and richness of life.

Emily Dickinson, in one of her poems, speaks of that first morning after the death of a loved one when so many things have changed and there is a new condition presented:

> The Bustle in a house
> The Morning after Death
> Is solemnest of industries
> Enacted upon Earth.
>
> The Sweeping up the Heart
> And putting Love away
> We shall not want to use again
> Until Eternity.[28]

This poem tells us of a moving and familiar experience among the members of the Cancer Family. Yet I see in these words another meaning beyond the activities of the household the morning after death. The morning *after* death does not quite concern me as much as the morning *before* death, of the time in which we contemplate what we are and where we are in the experience of life. I cannot quite escape the feeling that human beings come close to some kind of eternal insight when they discover that being worthy of life is of infinitely greater value than just possessing life. Robert S. DeRopp in his book *Drugs and the Mind* speaks of mental illness in the following way. "Madness," he writes, "severs the strongest bonds that hold human beings together. It separates husband from wife, mother from child. It is death without death's finality and without death's dignity." [29]

I quote DeRopp here not so much because he speaks

of a certain societal attitude toward mental illness, but because he lifts up an important insight about death. This quotation speaks of death's dignity. We can see here that we do possess the capacity to confront death with dignity just as we have the capacity to confront life with dignity. Whatever sickness may do to the body, whatever use may need to be made of pain-killing drugs, the attitude of the mind toward that illness, and toward death, is crucial for the experience. There is open to us the determination of how and in what name we are to experience death. I find this fact so real and so open to full possibility that I sometimes wonder why death is still so dreaded. When we have lived well we may die well. That is more than a play on words. What we say about death, the attitudes we have toward ourselves, our existence, toward persons around us, the manner in which we speak of our own possible death, is all a part of the freedom given us to choose the manner in which we move from life to death.

Paul Tillich, in a sermon entitled "The Eternal Now," writes:

> As men we are aware of the eternal to which we belong and from which we are estranged by the bondage of time.[30]

The prospect of death may help release us from this "bondage of time." Contemplating the death that may very well overtake us we are suddenly thrust into a new freedom of the spirit that is timeless. I believe this so strongly, and I have seen it manifested in the lives of so many persons around me, that I have come to feel the truth of it more and more with the passing of the years. In Emily Dickinson's sense there comes about in the human heart a bustle of gathering up the real things of one's possessions, a gathering about one of the prized things, the cherished thoughts, memories, victories, and joys, the things that gave substance to life. At the prospect of death we may bring these things into the open meadows of our vision. There we see them with new appreciation and tenderness. We gather loved ones around us and draw from them resources for life's refreshment. We reach out to collect the best things of life and to incorporate them into our new sense of what is of value. We may very well see a whole new working of the ways of the spiritual life and find the place for the power of that dimension. There is a bustle of the spirit that grows rather than diminishes in the face of death.

One of the open windows through which the breezes of newfound freedom from time may blow, in the prospect of death, is that of honesty with persons. There is much dishonesty about death just as there is dishonesty about life. Doctors hide facts from patients, patients refuse to talk about themselves to family members, and family members enter into an agreement that they will not talk about the illness. Outwardly there reigns a spirit of unanimity, but inwardly there is sometimes a great hunger to face things more openly. This conspiracy of silence is likely to be hard on both patient and family. When a patient learns that death may be inevitable he and his entire family may pretend something else. Often everyone acts as if the patient were to live forever when each person knows quite well that he will not. The pretense sometimes relieves the anxiety of the witnesses but it may also isolate persons from one another at precisely the time when there should be a drawing together. As one woman confided to her pastor: "My family doesn't talk to me. It is as if I were already dead. They won't even say good-by."

All this can be avoided in those moments when death becomes something to be talked about, faced, thought through, considered, and shared. My own experience is that when this is done, even though the beginning steps are often painful and hazardous, a new freedom from old feelings and hesitations is gained and assurance is provided.

These are the things I believe about death and dying. If we are to die, we may choose exactly how and in what name we are to experience death. Our death may be a victory for ourselves and for the conquest of all that hinders and causes us to feel cheated because death comes. It may very well present us with fulfillment rather than emptiness. Whether or not this is so in any individual situation depends entirely on how quickly we begin the process of meeting death squarely and gathering around us the resources that make death the victim and not the victor. Death becomes our victory when we choose to be filled with the spirit of thanksgiving and peace rather than with the spirit of despair or regret. We have the remarkable power to choose.

William Cullen Bryant was speaking to each one of us in this experience of death's possibilities when he wrote in "Thanatopsis":

> So live, that when thy summons comes to join
> The innumerable caravan, which moves
> To that mysterious realm, where each shall take
> His chamber in the silent halls of death,
> Thou go not, like the quarry-slave at night,
> Scourged to his dungeon, but, sustained and soothed
> By an unfaltering trust, approach thy grave,
> Like one who wraps the drapery of his couch
> About him, and lies down to pleasant dreams.[31]

Chapter 8

LIFE

WE COME NOW TO THE END of our journey through the world of cancer. We are novices in this journey, of course. I would use the term "pilgrim" here to denote those of us who travel along this way. We have not been this way before and we are often unsure of our footing. When cancer comes to us, or to a loved one, we enter into an entirely new experience. Not all the experience of others who have suffered before us, not all the books, advice, or personal testimonies of others can be of much help to us when we face it in our own lives. When the time for facing comes, we become pilgrims of a sort, journeymen, adventurers—until healing, remission, or death prevails.

In this book we have discovered some new trails in our pilgrimage. We have scaled a mountain or two of hope, have seen the lower valleys of cancer's grim toll, have thrashed around, so to speak, in some of the underbrush of statistics and scientific terms. Yet always we have seen the sunlight shining through the trees, and our path has not been entirely in darkness. For that, at least, we can be grateful.

Now, a final word. I speak to my fellow Family members. Whatever it is we are caused to do or endure in our experience of cancer, it remains for us to affirm life even though it be in the midst of the possibility of death. After all, if you can read this book, you are still alive. We cannot avoid living. Furthermore, if we are wise, we will let our adversities act upon us in such a way that our lives are enriched, not darkened, by those adversities. Edwin Markham set this out for us in his "Victory in Defeat." He wrote:

> Defeat may serve as well as victory
> To shake the soul and let the glory out.
> When the great oak is straining in the wind,
> The boughs drink in new beauty, and the trunk
> Sends down a deeper root on the windward side.
> Only the soul that knows the mighty grief
> Can know the mighty rapture. Sorrows come
> To stretch our spaces in the heart for joy.[32]

We are alive! Whatever has happened to us, or around us, we are alive now. There is no reason for us not to make that an experience of quality. Our days may be numbered if we are a cancer patient. We cannot be wholly sure about that. We may suffer pain even while we read this book. We may suffer for someone else close to us. Whatever the case may be, it need not detour us from making something out of the experience and out of ourselves as we move through the experience. From a hospital bed, from a wheelchair, from fear and grief and distress, we may make life an affirmation as did Alan Paton in his *Cry, the Beloved Country,* that great and haunting novel of South Africa. After writing of the pain and tragedy of so many innocent people, Paton says:

> The great valley of the Umzimkulu is still in darkness, but the light will come there. Ndotsheni is still in dark-

ness, but the light will come there also. For it is in the
dawn that has come, as it has come for a thousand
centuries, never failing. But when that dawn will come, of
our emancipation, from the fear of bondage and the
bondage of fear, why, that is a secret.[33]

Is this naïve? I do not think so. It is but a step from
this poetic expression of a truth about human endurance
to something that Ann Nietzke wrote recently. In speaking of our temptation to take the easy way out, to avoid
the pain and the confrontations of life, to disengage
ourselves from hard truth and from the necessity of doing
what must be done, she says:

> The price [we] pay for avoiding the pain of being fully
> alive is that [we] are excluded from the pleasure of it
> as well.[34]

What is said here is that the pain of human experience,
whether that pain be physical suffering, heartache, or
some other form of distress, is the price we pay for the
privilege of being fully alive. To be pain-free is to be half
dead, if not dead altogether. Few would choose that
consciously. Our pain is a symbol of our being alive,
and there is always, in the scheme of things, a price to
be paid for that fact.

Recently a play opened on Broadway called *To
Live Another Summer, To Pass Another Winter*. This
play is a musical interpretation of the lengthy history of
the Jewish people. It is a play that has boisterous singing, dancing, and considerable merrymaking, together
with dialogue that reflects the Jewish experience over the
centuries. Through persecution, torment, exile, and deprivation the Jewish people have managed somehow to
hang on, to pass through their successive times of
troubles, and to endure. The key to that endurance, ac-

cording to the play, is not so much any profound sense of history on the part of the Jewish people, certainly no particular ability to probe into the future for some disclosed or revealed destiny. The key to that endurance is simply a tenacity on the part of the Jewish people, a determination to go from one day to the next, from one season to the next, in thanksgiving for being alive. If fate will allow them to live just another summer and to pass just another winter, then perhaps, after all, things will be better.

That is a remarkable philosophy and one which we might well envy. We might also very well practice it in the experience of cancer. Whatever we are to be given in the future of that experience, whatever we might be given or whatever might be taken away—if we can but live for one more summer of appreciation for some good or some gift, and if we can pass just one more winter of trial or lack, we will have shown something magnificent about the power of life and our love for it.

As for the Jewish people in the long history of their struggle to endure, so also for us there is the sure knowledge that life works for our good. Paul the apostle put it in his own peculiar way:

> We are handicapped on all sides, but we are never frustrated; we are puzzled, but never in despair. We are persecuted, but we never have to stand it alone; we may be knocked down but we are never knocked out! . . . We are always facing death, but this means that you know more and more of life. (II Cor. 4:8, 9, 12; Phillips.)

We need to appreciate the continuing truth of this ancient wisdom.

NOTES

1. *Youth Looks at Cancer*, booklet published by the American Cancer Society, 1960, p. 5.

2. From pamphlet *Cigarette Smoking and Lung Cancer*, American Cancer Society, 1965, Q. 1.

3. *Ibid.*, Q. 1, 24.

4. For this information, and for most of the statistical data used elsewhere in this book, I am indebted to a pamphlet, *'74 Cancer Facts and Figures*, published by the American Cancer Society. Grateful acknowledgment is made to the Society for permission to quote from this publication.

5. *Ibid.*, p. 8.

6. Statistics are for the year 1964–1965. Segi, Mitsuo, *et al., Cancer Mortality for Selected Sites, No. 5*, reported in *'72 Cancer Facts and Figures* (American Cancer Society), p. 8.

7. Reported in Lauren V. Ackerman and Juan A. del Regato, *Cancer—Diagnosis, Treatment and Prognosis*, 4th ed. (C. V. Mosby Company, 1970), p. 849.

8. *The Merck Manual of Diagnosis and Therapy*, 11th ed. (Merck & Co., Inc., 1966), p. 151.

9. Turnley Walker, *Rise Up and Walk*, p. 35.

10. C. S. Lewis, *A Grief Observed*, p. 7.

11. Charles W. Wahl, "The Fear of Death," in *The Meaning of Death*, Herman Feifel, ed. (McGraw-Hill Publishing Company, Inc., 1959), p. 28.

12. D. H. Lawrence, "The Ship of Death," from *Master Poems of the English Language*, Oscar Williams, ed. (Simon & Schuster, Inc., 1966), p. 907.

13. Alice and A. Dudley Ward, *I Remain Unvanquished*, pp. 67-68.

14. Reported in *Cancer*, Vol. XXIX, No. 4 (April, 1972).

15. Karl Menninger, *Man Against Himself* (Harcourt Brace & Company, Inc., 1938), p. 449.

16. *The Healing Church* (The Tübingen Consultation 1964). World Council Studies No. 3 (Geneva: World Council of Churches, 1965), p. 45.

17. John Howard Griffin, "The Terrain of Physical Pain" in Alan Paton *et al.*, *Creative Suffering: The Ripple of Hope* (Pilgrim Press, 1970), p. 32.

18. Alan Paton, "Why Suffering?" in Paton, ed., *Creative Suffering*, p. 15.

19. Michel Quoist, *Prayers*, tr. by Angus M. Forsyth and Ann Marie de Commaille (Sheed & Ward, Inc., 1963), p. 144.

20. Albert Camus, *Resistance, Rebellion and Death*, tr. by Justin O'Brien (Alfred A. Knopf, Inc., 1961), p. 272.

21. Ward, *I Remain Unvanquished*, p. 62.

22. James D. Bryden, *Letters to Mark on God's Relation to Human Suffering* (Harper & Brothers, 1953), p. 134.

23. White, ed., *Dialogue in Medicine and Theology*, p. 68.

24. Paul Tournier, *The Meaning of Persons*, p. 111.

25. For evidence of some of these verifications see Ambrose and Olga Worrall, *The Gift of Healing: A Personal Story of Spiritual Therapy* (Harper & Row, Publishers, Inc., 1965), pp. 142-151.

26. *The Last Whole Earth Catalog* (Random House, Inc., 1971). The quotation is from *Energy Flow in Biology*, by Harold J. Morowitz (Academic Press, 1968).

27. Maria H. Nagy, "The Child's View of Death," from *The Meaning of Death*, Herman Feifel, ed. (McGraw-Hill Book Co., Inc., 1959), p. 90.

28. *The Complete Poems of Emily Dickinson,* ed. by Thomas H. Johnson (Little, Brown & Company, 1960), p. 489.

29. Robert S. DeRopp, *Drugs and the Mind* (St. Martin's Press, 1957), pp. 167-168.

30. Paul Tillich, "The Eternal Now," from his *The Eternal Now* (Charles Scribner's Sons, 1963), p. 123.

31. William Cullen Bryant, "Thanatopsis," *The Home Book of Verse*, arr. by B. E. Stevenson, Vol. II (Henry Holt & Company, 1912), p. 3444. Used by permission of Holt, Rinehart and Winston, Inc.

32. Edwin Markham, "Victory in Defeat," *Masterpieces of Religious Verse*, ed. by James D. Morrison (Harper & Brothers, 1948), p. 292.

33. Alan Paton, *Cry, the Beloved Country* (London: Jonathan Cape, Ltd., 1948), p. 253.

34. Ann Nietzke, in *Saturday Review*, Vol. LV, No. 35 (Aug. 26, 1972), p. 34.

BIBLIOGRAPHY

Selections for this bibliography were made primarily on the basis of their ability to speak to the matter of suffering or healing. In addition, I have included materials relating to the disease of cancer and the place of the human spirit in that experience.

American Cancer Society, *'74 Cancer Facts and Figures.*

Brown, Norman O., *Life Against Death.* Random House, Inc., 1959.

DeVries, Peter, *Blood of the Lamb* (Chs. 12-16). Little, Brown & Company, 1962.

Frank, Anne, *The Diary of a Young Girl,* tr. by B. M. Mooyaart-Doubleday. Doubleday & Company, Inc., 1967.

Lambourne, Robert A., *Community, Church and Healing.* London: Darton, Longman & Todd, Ltd., 1963.

Lewis, C. S., *A Grief Observed.* The Seabury Press, 1961.

Martin, Bernard, *The Healing Ministry in the Church.* John Knox Press, 1960.

Paton, Alan, *et al., Creative Suffering: The Ripple of Hope.* Pilgrim Press, 1970.

Sandoz, Mari, *Cheyenne Autumn.* McGraw-Hill Book Company, Inc., 1953.

Tournier, Paul, *The Meaning of Persons,* tr. by Edwin Hudson. Harper & Brothers, 1957.

Walker, Turnley, *Rise Up and Walk*. E. P. Dutton & Co., Inc., 1950.

Ward, Alice and A. Dudley, *I Remain Unvanquished*. Abingdon Press, 1970.

Weatherhead, Leslie, *Why Do Men Suffer?* Abingdon Press, 1936.

White, Dale., ed., *Dialogue in Medicine and Theology*. Abingdon Press, 1968.

Wise, Carroll A., *Psychiatry and the Bible*. Harper & Brothers, 1956.